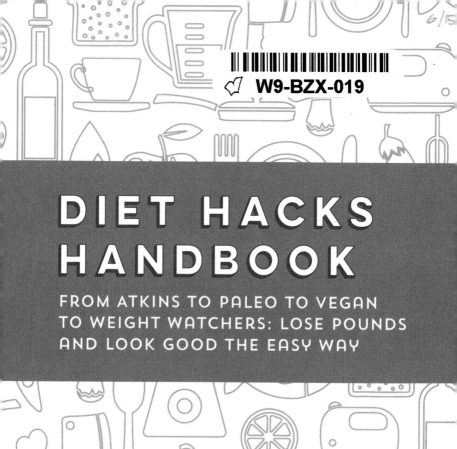

DIET HACKS HANDBOOK

FROM ATKINS TO PALEO TO VEGAN
TO WEIGHT WATCHERS: LOSE POUNDS
AND LOOK GOOD THE EASY WAY

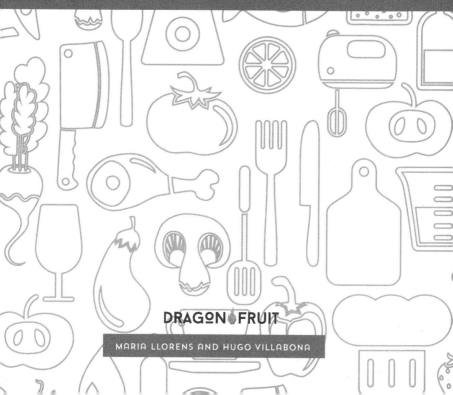

DRAGON FRUIT

MARIA LLORENS AND HUGO VILLABONA

DISCLAIMER

Welcome to Diet Hacks Handbook, the definitive breakdown of diets, trends, programs, food pyramids, and all things caloric. We have compiled observations, Google-centric analytics, research and opinions to inform and educate you as much as possible about all things dietary. However, and we cannot stress this enough, please, please consult your healthcare professional, doctor, mom, next door neighbor or the nursing student you see on the bus every morning before you make any drastic change in your daily regimen.

There is no guarantee that Diet Hacks will in fact hack your diet, result in weight-loss or improve your health...although, we like to think that it will. We hope you enjoy, read, attempt and even perfect our diet suggestions. But remember, we warned you.

Research Disclaimer: All fitness statistics were obtained via social media outlets, weight loss forums and online dieting communities. Participants were asked to state their age, weight, gender, the diet they had attempted, their results, if they would recommend daily exercise and if they would do the diet again. All other factors of the individuals were kept anonymous. Not all diets garnered the same ratio of participants and comments, therefore, some numbers were taken at a percentage and then averaged out to a sample-size of 100 participants.

"God made food, the devil the cooks."
- James Joyce

CONTENTS

PREFACE   07

CHAPTER 1 // Diets   08

South Beach Diet   11
Atkins Diet   15
Paleo Diet   19
The Zone Diet   23
Volumetrics   27
Raw Food Diet   31
Vegetarian & Vegan Diets   35
DASH Diet   39
TLC Diet   43
Traditional Asian Diet   48
Macrobiotic Diet   52
Mediterranean Diet   55

CHAPTER 2 // Programs   58

Weight Watchers   61
Jenny Craig   64
Nutrisystem   67
Slim-Fast   70
Biggest Loser   73
HerbaLife   76

CHAPTER 3 // Breaking Down the Food Pyramid   78

Nutrition Basics   81
Top 10 Diet and Health Myths   90
Make Vegetables Work for You   95

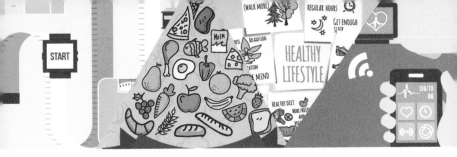

CHAPTER 4 // Diet Hacks   99

How to Diet Without Dieting   102
How to Eat Your Veggies   106
How to Stick to Your Diet   110
How to Diet While Vacationing   114
How to Diet Unconventionally   116

CHAPTER 5 // Digitize Your Diet   119

Counting Calories   122
Planning Meals   125
Track Your Weight   128
Know What's in Your Food   130

Sources   132
Image Credits   138

PREFACE

We live in a world where fitness trends, diets, and what we just ate are as pertinent to our social circles as selfies are to Instagram. It's the age of information and this excess of knowledge has sparked a health movement. With films like *Super-Size Me* and *Food, Inc.* leading the way, healthy lifestyles have become less about the numbers and more about pop culture. From eating organically to learning about gluten-free foods to following Beyoncé's exercise routine, the 21st century has reached a new level of healthy living that is borderline obsessive, but in a good way. The healthy lifestyle of this millennium is constantly evolving on morning shows, the Food Network, magazines and infomercials. It feels like this complicated and rarely applied level of knowledge that we want to keep up with, but can't. That is where we come in. We feel we can simplify, streamline, facilitate, and convey all things about diets in a convenient manner.

We aren't focused on a particular reason to eat better. Whether you're in it for weight-loss or lower blood pressure, our goal is to give you simple ideas and solutions to practice a healthier diet.

Everyone at one point or another will struggle with their health in some way. So don't overthink it, don't stress too much. Just take it at pace--remember, we're no experts--just use the icons and information to guide you. The next time you're considering losing a couple of pounds or maybe adding a few bulky muscles, you'll know where to start.

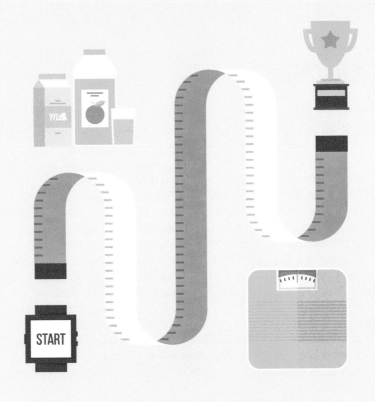

CHAPTER 1 //
DIETS

How to Use This Section

Our first chapter weighs the pros and cons of 12 popular diets. You've heard of these in the news, on talk shows, and from your health-nut friends. But should you buy into them? In each section, we explain the diets' various goals with these components:

The Hack Sheet

The icons at the top are a quick guide to the foods that are recommended for the diet plan.

By the Numbers

The charts and statistics are the result of our small survey of health and fitness fanatics. They measure the weight loss effectiveness of each diet.

Who? What? How?

These sections describe the origin of each diet, the concept behind it, and the steps that it requires.

Pros and Cons

We offer our ideas on the overall benefits of the diet and how difficult it is to follow.

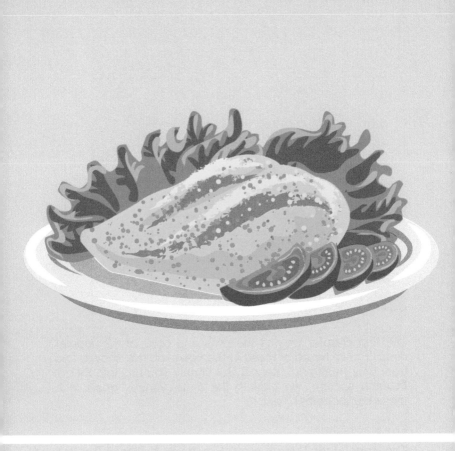

Diet //
South Beach Diet

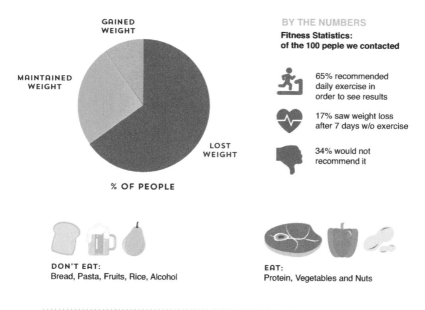

GAINED
WEIGHT

MAINTAINED
WEIGHT

LOST
WEIGHT

% OF PEOPLE

BY THE NUMBERS

**Fitness Statistics:
of the 100 peple we contacted**

65% recommended
daily exercise in
order to see results

17% saw weight loss
after 7 days w/o exercise

34% would not
recommend it

DON'T EAT:
Bread, Pasta, Fruits, Rice, Alcohol

EAT:
Protein, Vegetables and Nuts

Who made it?

The South Beach Diet was started by a dietician named Marie Almon and a cardiologist named Arthur. It turns out he has his office in Miami Beach, hence the name: South Beach Diet.

What's it for?

 It is the diet with the snazziest name. From a marketing standpoint, it screams summer, bathing suits, beaches, relaxation and everything that a diet isn't.

It is the claim here is that it is not a diet, but rather a healthy eating plan which modifies the overall balance of the foods you consume to inspire weight loss and a healthy lifestyle.

The concept is centered on eliminating what they refer to as "bad" carbs. Simply put, carbs are labeled as either "good" or "bad" based on their glycemic index and glycemic load. In layman's terms, foods with a high glycemic index are said to increase blood sugar for a longer period faster, thus resulting in a bigger appetite, bigger portions of food and bigger waistlines.

A closer look into the diet will show that it informs the user on fats, fiber, and whole grains and how they too can be categorized as either "good" or "bad."

How it Works
The diet is broken down into 3 phases:

Phase 1 revolves around eliminating the foods that cause cravings. It's basically a strict regimen of lean proteins, water, unsaturated fats, nuts and seeds.

Phase 2 is initiated by re-introducing a few of the eliminated foods from phase 1 back into your daily intake.

Phase 3 kicks in once you have reached a healthy weight. At this point simply apply what you learned in phases 1 and 2 to limit "bad" carbs and maintain a healthy size.

Pros

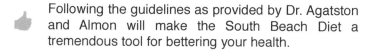

Following the guidelines as provided by Dr. Agatston and Almon will make the South Beach Diet a tremendous tool for bettering your health.

You can reduce your waistline and improve your health while still being able to enjoy some great foods.

Cons

If you don't follow the plan as directed, you can run into some major risks.

According to the Mayo Clinic, severely restricting your carbs can result in problems from ketosis. Basically, ketosis occurs when you remove carbs entirely from your diet and you don't have enough sugar (glucose) for energy.

As a result of this lack of pep, your body will break down the extra fat, causing ketones to build up in your body. Side effects from ketosis can include nausea, headache, mental fatigue, bad breath, and sometimes dehydration and dizziness.

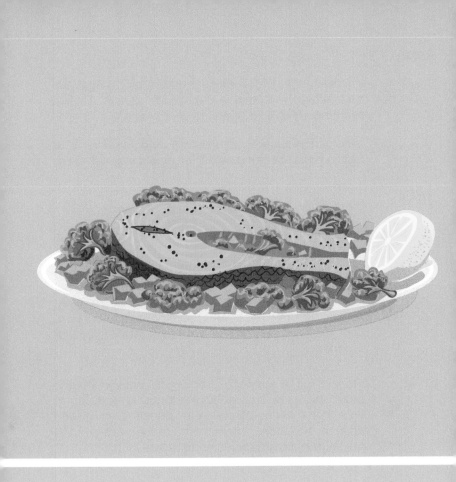

Diet //
Atkins Diet

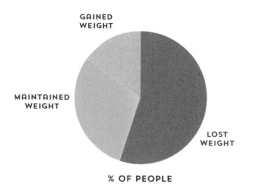

GAINED WEIGHT

MAINTAINED WEIGHT

LOST WEIGHT

% OF PEOPLE

**Fitness Statistics:
of the 100 peple we contacted**

 55% recommended
daily exercise in
order to see results

 11% saw weight loss
after 7 days w/o exercise

 54% would not
recommend it

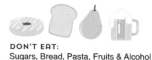

DON'T EAT:
Sugars, Bread, Pasta, Fruits & Alcohol

EAT:
Protein, Vegetables and Cheese

Who made it?

The Atkins Diet goes back to the 1960s. Dr. Alfred W. Pennington published an article in the *Journal of the American Medical Association* discussing the concept of removing all starches and sugars from meals. Dr. Robert Atkins, an overweight cardiologist, tweaked the formula to create his diet plan. Atkins felt that carbs were the bad guys. Through his extensive research, he found that carbs caused the body to create an abundance of the hormone insulin: hyperinsulinism.

What's it for?

It is a very controversial diet. Think of it as the legalization of marijuana in the diet world. Many doctors, nutritionists and other experts have expressed their concerns that the diet is an oversimplification of the metabolic processes.

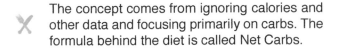 The concept comes from ignoring calories and other data and focusing primarily on carbs. The formula behind the diet is called Net Carbs.

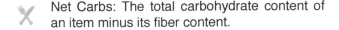 Net Carbs: The total carbohydrate content of an item minus its fiber content.

How it Works:
The diet is broken down into 4 phases:

Phase 1 is the strictest. This phase requires you to eliminate almost all carbohydrates from your diet, consuming no more than 20 grams of net carbs per day of which the majority should be from vegetables. During this phase you should consume protein at every meal, via meat, eggs and cheese. You don't need to eliminate oils and fats, but you do need to eliminate fruits, baked goods, breads, pastas, grains, nuts and alcohol for roughly two weeks.

Phase 2 keeps the minimum of 12-15 grams of net carbs via vegetables. You are still not allowed to have sugar. You can, however, add a few fruits (e.g. berries), as well as some nuts and seeds, so long as you are losing weight. The phase comes to a close after a 10 pound loss.

Phase 3 begins with a gradual increase in your menu selection, including fruits, starchy veggies and whole grains. Minimum carbs, like 10 grams, can be added, but if you gain weight at any point, they must be cut out completely. This phase ends when you would like it to. It is basically the phase of minimum loss while maintaining a healthy body.

Phase 4. Once you're happy and healthy, you can introduce the bad foods, like beer and bread, so long as you don't gain weight.

Pros

Following the guidelines as provided by Dr. Atkins will probably result in some weight loss, although even they claim that the initial loss (up to 15 pounds in a week) can be mainly water weight.

Overall, increasing veggies and removing sugars is never a bad thing.

Cons

If you don't follow the plan as directed, you can run into some major risks. According to the Mayo Clinic, headaches, weakness, dizziness and fatigue are concerns to consider when starting this diet.

And as stated before, there are dietary professionals and doctors who have voiced strong negative opinions on the diet.

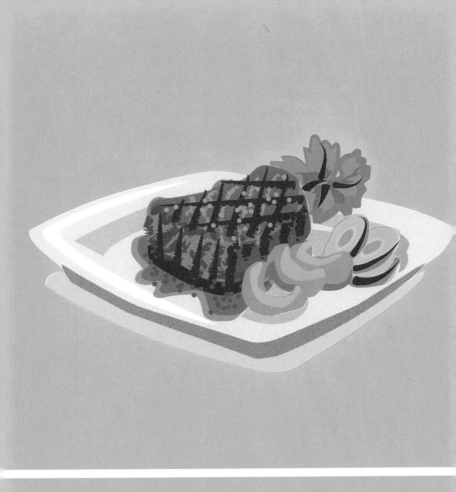

**Diet //
Paleo Diet**

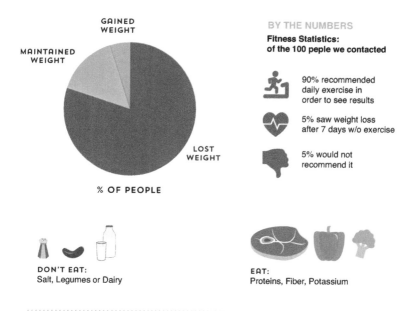

GAINED WEIGHT

MAINTAINED WEIGHT

LOST WEIGHT

% OF PEOPLE

BY THE NUMBERS

**Fitness Statistics:
of the 100 peple we contacted**

90% recommended daily exercise in order to see results

5% saw weight loss after 7 days w/o exercise

5% would not recommend it

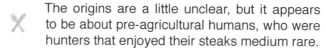

DON'T EAT:
Salt, Legumes or Dairy

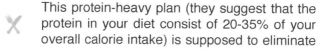

EAT:
Proteins, Fiber, Potassium

Who made it?

Tyrannosaurus Rex...just kidding. No, actually in 1975 there was a book about the Stone Age and the nutrition of our ancestors. That book inspired a research project, which resulted in a study published in the *New England Journal of Medicine*. That article made its way to Loren Cordain, Ph.D and he branded it, applied it, sold it, and did just about everything he could to get it into the world.

What's it for?

✗ The origins are a little unclear, but it appears to be about pre-agricultural humans, who were hunters that enjoyed their steaks medium rare.

✗ This protein-heavy plan (they suggest that the protein in your diet consist of 20-35% of your overall calorie intake) is supposed to eliminate the unnatural food that we consume while improving your body's health with more fiber, good fats and potassium.

Processed foods, milk, alcohol, salt, etc. are all items that go against the dining hunter's creed These foods are essentially prohibited from your diet in order to restore your body to its pre-farmer form.

How it Works:

The diet isn't about phases and nonsensical charts. It's pretty straight forward. Eat this. Don't eat that. Results will vary, but ultimately, the Paleo people feel that this more natural origins diet will improve your overall health, which will lead your body to naturally eliminate any excess.

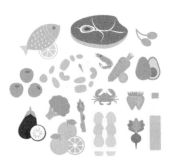

EAT:
- Grass-produced meats
- Fish/seafood
- Fresh fruits & veggies
- Eggs
- Nuts & seeds
- Healthful oils
  (olive, walnut, flaxseed, macadamia, avocado, coconut)

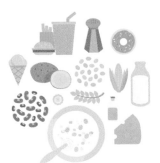

DON'T EAT:
- Cereal grains
- Legumes (including peanuts)
- Dairy
- Refined sugar
- Potatoes
- Processed foods
- Salt
- Refined vegetable oils

Pros

 You get to eat meat.

 The diet offers some strong claims and the people we contacted for feedback loved it more than any other diet.

 However, take that with a grain of salt, as most of the people we spoke to were already very healthy and fit. So their initial goal was not to lose 10, 20, 30 pounds, but instead to be a leaner, fitter version of an already healthy looking body.

Cons

 Based on our research, it is not really a diet for major weight loss (more than 5 pounds or so). It is more for people looking to change their routines.

It can result in weight loss, but the people we contacted via Men's Health said that without exercise, the diet is just a funky way of consuming large amounts of protein while claiming to be on a diet.

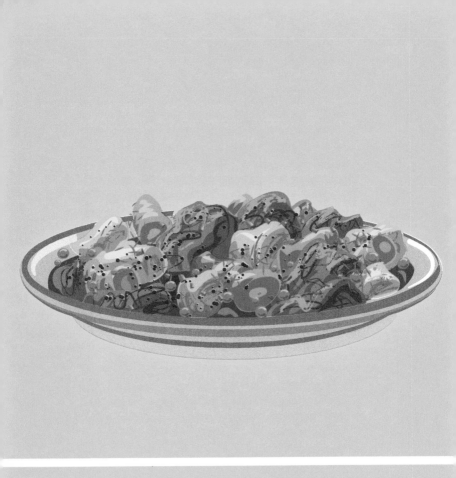

Diet //
The Zone Diet

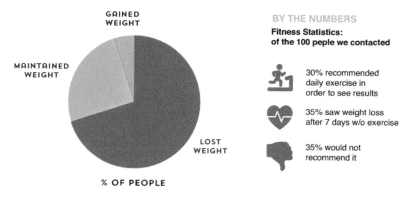

GAINED
WEIGHT

MAINTAINED
WEIGHT

LOST
WEIGHT

% OF PEOPLE

Fitness Statistics:
of the 100 pepple we contacted

 30% recommended
daily exercise in
order to see results

 35% saw weight loss
after 7 days w/o exercise

 35% would not
recommend it

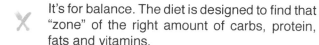

DON'T EAT:
White bread, white rice, and
other processed products.

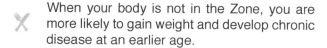

EAT:
Colorful veggies, proteins, dairies,
fruits and nuts.

Who made it?

Biochemist Barry Sears created the Zone Diet as a way to stabilize blood sugar levels, lower inflammation and create an overall healthier life. There are rumors online that his main objective behind the Zone Diet was to reduce his chances of dying from cardiac arrest as many of the men in his family had died from heart complications.

What's it for?

X   It's for balance. The diet is designed to find that "zone" of the right amount of carbs, protein, fats and vitamins.

X   When your body is not in the Zone, you are more likely to gain weight and develop chronic disease at an earlier age.

The overall concept of this diet, according to the website, is that "The Zone" is as real as the air we breathe. They call it a physiological condition, where the cellular inflammation is not too low to the point that you can't fight off infection, but not so high that the body begins to attack itself.

How it Works:
This diet wants you to eat less white (white bread, white rice, white pasta, and white potatoes).

Here's how to do it:

1. If you can eliminate these whites from your diet then you'll have less cellular inflammation.

2. This anti-inflammatory zone is meant to be reached via a strict diet and then sustained for a prolonged period (ideally, your entire life).

3. Once you're in the Zone (sounds ridiculous, but work with it), you can begin to control the expression of inflammatory genes.

4. This results in a healthier heart and, in turn, a healthier body.

5. The Zone Diet can be pushed to another level by anti-inflammatory supplements, such as omega-3 fatty acids and polyphenols. Like the Paleo diet, this is less a stage diet and more of a lifestyle.

Pros

 It is very easy to start, follow and finish.

 There are not a lot of rules and you have a hearty menu to pick from since the diet wants you to have a nutritional balance.

 Sticking to the Zone diet may help you lose weight and lower your risk of heart disease, according to a study published in the *Journal of the American Medical Association.*

Cons

 The meals within the Zone diet should have a 40 to 30 to 30 (protein, carbs, oils) macronutrient breakdown, which many found to be exhausting to track.

 Also, because the diet tends to be very low in calories, many of the participants complained about being hungry throughout the day.

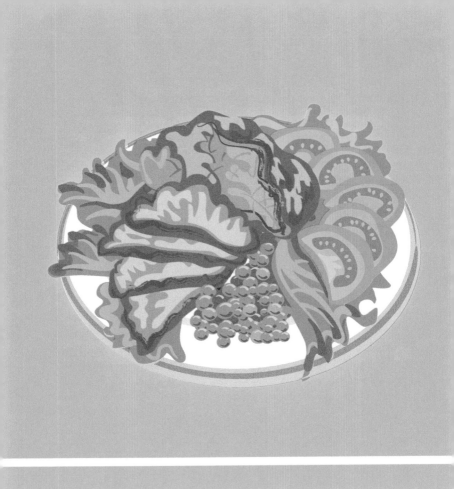

Diet //
Volumetrics

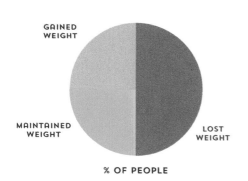

GAINED
WEIGHT

MAINTAINED
WEIGHT

LOST
WEIGHT

% OF PEOPLE

Fitness Statistics:
of the 100 peple we contacted

80% recommended
daily exercise in
order to see results

10% saw weight loss
after 7 days w/o exercise

75% would not
recommend it

EAT:
Just about anything. From healthy veggies
and fruits to fries and cake.

Who made it?

Dr. Barbara Rolls, professor of Biobehavioral Health at Penn State University, began this diet with the idea of losing weight while eating what you love. Going against the norm of diets based on deprivation, Volumetrics guides the individual to find healthy foods that they can eat lots of while still losing weight.

What's it for?

It's for energy. Dr. Rolls argues that instead of tracking your calorie intake, you should track the energy density of the foods you consume.

Energy density? The Live Strong foundation labels energy density as a ratio: calories per gram. Basically, foods that are lower on the energy density totem pole are bulkier, so they carry less calories.

These bulky foods are high in fiber and water content, so after you eat them you feel pretty full for a long time.

How it Works:

This diet is all about a strict game plan on a fairly flexible menu. The good doctor separates foods into four categories:

Category 1: Freedom in the form of fruits, non-starchy vegetables (e.g. broccoli, tomatoes, mushrooms), and broth-based soups whenever you want them.

Category 2: Intelligent portions of whole grains (e.g. brown rice and whole wheat pasta), lean proteins, legumes, and low-fat dairy.

Category 3: The good stuff in small portions. Small breads, desserts, fat-free baked snacks, cheeses, and higher-fat meats.

Category 4: The really good stuff, but with a once-in-a-blue-moon mindset. Sparing portions of fried foods, candy, cookies, nuts, and fats.

You'll eat three meals, two snacks, and a dessert each day. Told you. Open menu, strict guidelines.

Pros

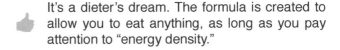

It's a dieter's dream. The formula is created to allow you to eat anything, as long as you pay attention to "energy density."

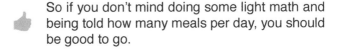

So if you don't mind doing some light math and being told how many meals per day, you should be good to go.

Cons

You can have beer....so that alone makes you question the diet's validity.

The truth is that Dr. Rolls has tremendous credentials and she isn't creating some revolution. At its core, Volumetrics is a lower calories, lower fat, lots of vegetables and fruits and a hint of "trust" diet.

The biggest con here is having enough self-control to handle the open menu.

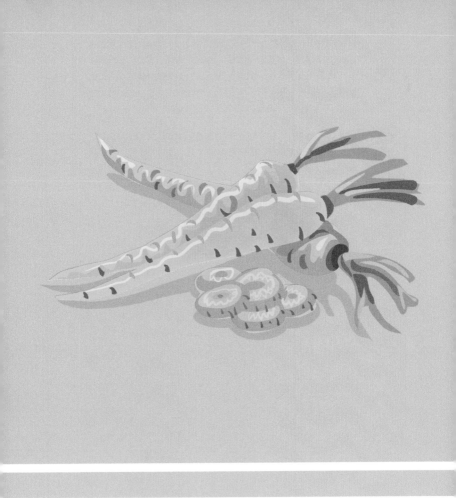

**Diet //
Raw Food Diet**

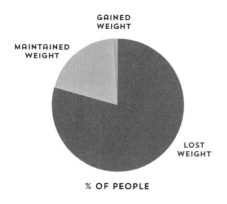

% OF PEOPLE

Fitness Statistics:
of the 100 peple we contacted

20% recommended
daily exercise in
order to see results

85% saw weight loss
after 7 days w/o exercise

5% would not
recommend it

DON'T EAT:
If it requires fire, leave it alone.

EAT:
If a bunny can eat it, so can you.
Think greens, fruits and uncooked.

Who made it?

Adam and Eve. Maybe. We don't really know. You see it doesn't have an origin outside of the dawn of time before man created fire and wheel. Historically, this diet has had its peaks during cultural phenomena, like a spike in interest during the gluten phase or when hipsters made being vegan and wearing sunglasses indoors popular.

What's it for?

The diet is very trendy and social media friendly. It's for people who want to be environmentally conscious while losing a few pounds.

It's not hard to grasp and you don't need to count calories or divide carbs by sugar while turning the sodium into an exponent. It's just: eat raw.

How it Works:
This diet is meant to be a natural instinct:

1. If you set your mind to focus on foods that never need to be cooked, foods that are completely unprocessed, mostly organic food, you'll adjust quickly.

2. Meals should consist of: raw fruits, veggies, nuts, seeds, and sprouted grains. There are differing opinions on consuming unpasteurized dairy foods, raw eggs and raw fish.

3. Cooking is generally defined by the diet as anything heated above 118 degrees. Prior to that, the food should retain its natural benefits.

4. You can use blenders, food processors, and dehydrators to prepare foods.

Pros

 You will most likely lose weight on this diet, since most raw foods are low in calories, fat, and sodium, while being very high in fiber.

 Another fantastic benefit to the Raw Food diet is that you get nutritional perks.

 Most of what you eat will be high in some vitamins, minerals, fiber, and phytochemicals.

Cons

 The drawback comes from the lifestyle. If you follow the diet and are very strict with it, you will definitely see results, but you will be lacking in protein, iron, calcium, and other vitamins and minerals.

 Excluding animal products / "cooked foods" from your diet may lead to having to take vitamin supplements and other health complications.

 So it is best to do further research as to what foods you can completely eliminate from your diet.

Diet //
Vegetarian & Vegan Diets

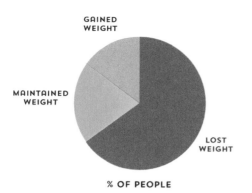

GAINED
WEIGHT

MAINTAINED
WEIGHT

LOST
WEIGHT

% OF PEOPLE

Fitness Statistics:
of the 100 peple we contacted

80% recommended
daily exercise in
order to see results

20% saw weight loss
after 7 days w/o exercise

5% would not
recommend it

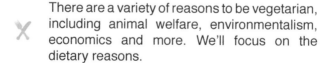

DON'T EAT:
Meat or foods made from meat
and meat by products.

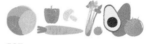

EAT:
Vegetables only.

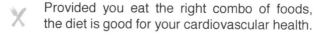

Who made it?

These have been around a while, probably since humans
settled down and created agriculture. The ancient Greek phi-
losopher Pythagoras, born in 570 B.C., promoted the virtues
of vegetarianism (though he may have eaten fish, making
him a pescatarian).

What's it for?

There are a variety of reasons to be vegetarian,
including animal welfare, environmentalism,
economics and more. We'll focus on the
dietary reasons.

It's likely you could lose weight on a vegetarian
diet. Research shows vegetarians have lower
body fat percentages and eat fewer calories
(while still feeling full).

Provided you eat the right combo of foods,
the diet is good for your cardiovascular health.

Simply being animal-free isn't enough (Oreos and Doritos are vegan, for instance).

Some research shows a balanced vegetarian diet can improve your mood, give you more energy, and help you avoid food-borne illnesses from meat and seafood.

How it Works :
There are actually a lot of different options for a more veggie-oriented diet:

1. **Vegan:** No meat, seafood, poultry, eggs, dairy or foods that contain these products.

2. **Lacto-vegetarian:** No meat, seafood, poultry or eggs. Milk, cheese, butter and other dairy products are okay to eat.

3. **Lacto-ovo vegetarian:** No meat, seafood, or poultry. Dairy and eggs are allowed.

4. **Ovo-vegetarian:** No meat, seafood, poultry or dairy products. Eggs are allowed.

5. **Pescatarian:** No meat or poultry, but seafood is allowed.

6. **Flexitarian:** Eat animal-based foods in small amounts or on special occasions.

Pros

👍 Better overall health and possible weight loss if healthy foods are consumed.

👍 Meals will be more filling and you'll be less hungry throughout the day.

👍 Many recipes and resources available.

👍 Restaurants are increasingly offering veggie-friendly options.

👍 Easily adapted to religious and dietary restrictions.

Cons

👎 Can be a difficult transition if you really enjoy meat and animal-based foods.

👎 Fresh vegetables, fruits, whole grains and organic products are often pricier than processed grains, sugar and snacks.

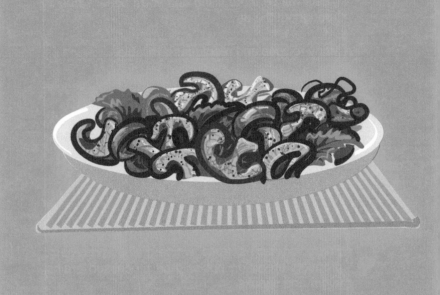

Diet //
The DASH Diet

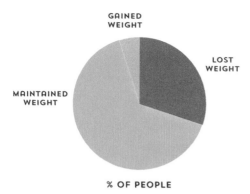

GAINED WEIGHT

LOST WEIGHT

MAINTAINED WEIGHT

% OF PEOPLE

BY THE NUMBERS

Fitness Statistics:
of the 100 peple we contacted

 65% recommended
daily exercise in
order to see results

 15% saw weight loss
after 7 days w/o exercise

 40% would not
recommend it

DON'T EAT:
Fast food and packaged high-sodium
foods, like chips, French fries, and cookies.

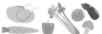

EAT:
Balanced diet, eat more vegetables
and other low-sodium foods.

Who made it?

DASH stands for Dietary Approaches to Stop Hypertension. The National Heart, Lung, and Blood Institute (NHLBI), created the diet based on their research studies that aimed to reduce heart disease and high blood pressure.

What's it for?

 DASH's claim is that a healthy eating pattern is key to bringing down high blood pressure along with your waistline.

 The diet focuses on "nutrients of concern" like potassium, calcium, protein and fiber. They're seen as crucial to fending off high blood pressure and Americans eat too few of them.

 You don't have to go nuts tracking nutrients, just eat more of the foods doctors say are good for you—fruits, veggies, whole grains and lean protein. Avoid those calorie-saturated snacks, sweets and red meat and you're good to go.

How it Works:
The diet focuses on these elements:

1.

Sodium levels. Depending on your health needs, you should be eating between 1,500 mg and 2,300 mg of sodium a day.

2.

A balanced diet. The standard food pyramid we grew up with still applies, but there's a new measure of healthy eating these days that's easier to visualize—the food plate. Fruits and vegetables should make up half of your intake, with fruits taking the smaller portion. The other half should be grains and protein, with protein taking up less space. A healthy sugar-free drink, like water or milk, is the last portion.

3.

Trim the treats. You don't have to abandon sweets altogether, but you should only have 5 or fewer a week. Try to choose fat-free or fruit-based snacks. Artificial sweeteners are okay in small amounts, but don't trade in water for diet soda.

Pros

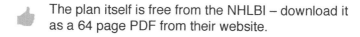 The plan itself is free from the NHLBI – download it as a 64 page PDF from their website.

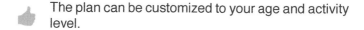 The plan can be customized to your age and activity level.

It's compatible with any other dietary restrictions – like vegetarian or gluten-free diets.

While not guaranteed, it's very likely that cutting unhealthy foods from your diet will lead to weight loss.

Cons

Processed, unhealthy foods are cheaper than fresh veggies and other healthy items.

Planning and cooking meals can often be time-consuming.

Cut down on party time: eating out and drinking alcohol have to be restricted to special occasions.

Diet //
The TLC Diet

TLC Diet

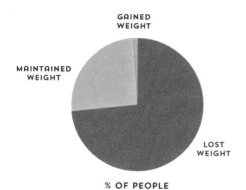

GAINED
WEIGHT

MAINTAINED
WEIGHT

LOST
WEIGHT

% OF PEOPLE

**Fitness Statistics:
of the 100 peple we contacted**

95% recommended
daily exercise in
order to see results

>1% saw weight loss
after 7 days w/o exercise

5% would not
recommend it

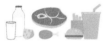

DON'T EAT:
**Avoid high saturated fat content, like
full-fat dairy, fatty meat and fried foods.**

EAT:
**More fruits, veggies, whole grains,
non-fat dairy, fish and skinless poultry.**

Who made it?

TLC, which stands for Therapeutic Life Changes, was created
by the National Institute of Health as part of their National Cholesterol Education Program. The recommendations are based
on research from medical trials and studies.

What's it for?

 The goal is to cut back significantly on your fat
intake to reduce the risk of high cholesterol and
cardiovascular disease without the need for
medication.

 Saturated fat—which comes from fatty meat,
high-fat dairy products and fried foods—is the
main focus.

 The diet claims you can cut your "bad" LDL
cholesterol by as much as 10 percent in less
than two months.

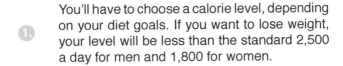

How it Works:

1. You'll have to choose a calorie level, depending on your diet goals. If you want to lose weight, your level will be less than the standard 2,500 a day for men and 1,800 for women.

2. Saturated fat will need to make up just 7 percent of daily calories. Refer to our handy chart on the next page for foods that you should avoid.

3. Cholesterol intake will need to go way, way down. As in 200 milligrams, or the amount in about 2 ounces of cheese.

4. Add more fiber to your diet if your cholesterol doesn't go down enough in six weeks. It blocks absorption of bad cholesterol in your body. Your best bet is by buying planet stanol or sterol supplements.

5. Instead of fatty foods, eat fruits, veggies, whole grains, non-fat dairy, fish and skinless poultry.

Pros

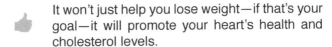

👍 It won't just help you lose weight—if that's your goal—it will promote your heart's health and cholesterol levels.

👍 It's not a fad diet. It's been researched by medical professionals.

👍 Guidelines are free and online, no purchase necessary. Your main resource is an 80-page manual called Your Guide to Lowering Your Cholesterol with TLC.

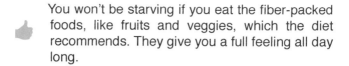 You won't be starving if you eat the fiber-packed foods, like fruits and veggies, which the diet recommends. They give you a full feeling all day long.

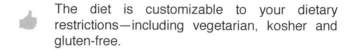 Your grocery bill should stay the same.

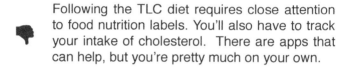 The diet is customizable to your dietary restrictions—including vegetarian, kosher and gluten-free.

Cons

Following the TLC diet requires close attention to food nutrition labels. You'll also have to track your intake of cholesterol. There are apps that can help, but you're pretty much on your own.

If you like buttery or greasy food, cheese, creamy sauces and fast food, this diet may require some adjustment. But there are solutions to keep your taste buds happy, like spices.

Food

8.5%
Regular cheese

5.9%
Pizza

5.8%
Grain-based desserts

5.6%
Dairy desserts

5.5%
Chicken & chicken mixed dishes

4.4%
Burgers

4.9%
Sausage, franks, bacon, & ribs

4.1%
Mexican mixed dishes

4.1%
Beef & beef mixed dishes

3.7%
Pasta & pasta dishes

3.9%
1%
Reduced fat milk

3.4%
100%
Whole milk

3.1%
Candy

2.9%
Butter

3.2%
Eggs & egg mixed dishes

2.0%
Fried white potatoes

2.4%
Potato/corn & other chips

2.1%
Nuts/seeds & nut/seed mixed dishes

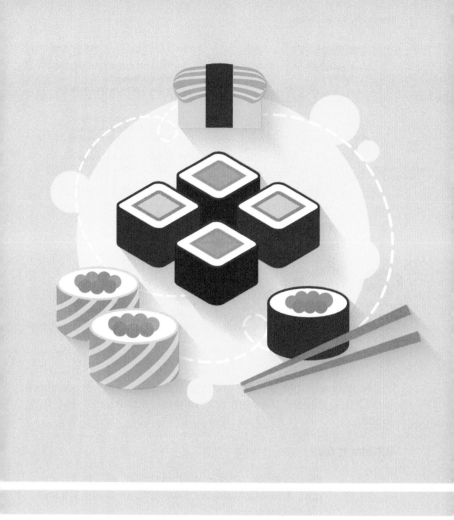

Diet //
The Traditional Asian Diet

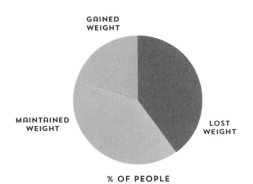

GAINED
WEIGHT

MAINTAINED
WEIGHT

LOST
WEIGHT

% OF PEOPLE

**Fitness Statistics:
of the 100 peple we contacted**

55% recommended
daily exercise in
order to see results

10% saw weight loss
after 7 days w/o exercise

30% would not
recommend it

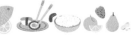

DON'T EAT:
Red meat should be eaten only monthly.
Eggs, poultry and sweets can be eaten
weekly. Fish and seafood can be eaten daily.

EAT:
Grains, fruits, vegetables, legumes and nuts
should be the primary component of daily meals.

There isn't a single "Asian" diet, but the typical diet in countries like China, Japan, Vietnam and others emphasizes less fatty foods.

What's it for?

 Proponents of the diet claim it will help you lose and maintain your weight, as well as avoid chronic disease.

 Studies have shown that people in Asian countries usually have lower rates of chronic diseases—cancer, heart disease and obesity—than Americans. They live longer, too.

 Researchers believe that this low-fat diet, with very little red meat and processed foods, is the reason for overall good health in Asian nations.

How it Works:

1. There isn't a single Asian diet, but the "Asian diet pyramid," developed by a Boston food think tank, is a good guide on how to start.

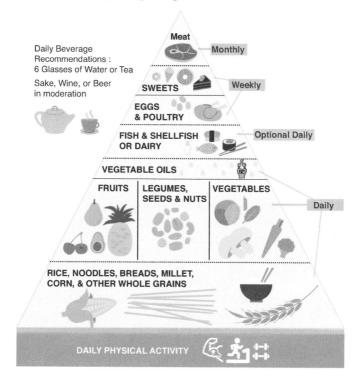

2. At the bottom of the pyramid are rice, noodles, and whole grains. Avoid processed grains.

3. Veggies, fruits, and anything else plant-related should be the second biggest component of the diet.

4. The diet is also hard on meat: red meat is only eaten monthly, while poultry and eggs are eaten weekly. Fish and other seafood can be eaten daily, but it's not required.

5. Sweets can be eaten weekly, but in smaller amounts.

6. Stay hydrated with 6 glasses of water or tea. Alcohol can be consumed in moderation.

Pros

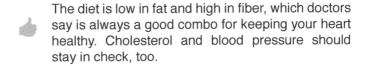 The diet is low in fat and high in fiber, which doctors say is always a good combo for keeping your heart healthy. Cholesterol and blood pressure should stay in check, too.

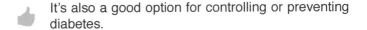 It's also a good option for controlling or preventing diabetes.

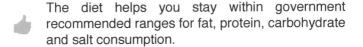 The diet helps you stay within government recommended ranges for fat, protein, carbohydrate and salt consumption.

Cons

If you don't like the idea of living off mostly rice, nuts, legumes, veggies and noodles, it may be difficult to adjust to this diet.

There are some decent resources online, but you'll probably have to invest in a recipe book or two.

Some items—fish, fresh produce and olive oil—can be on the pricey side. On the other hand, if you're currently spending a lot on meat, you'll cut that part of your grocery budget.

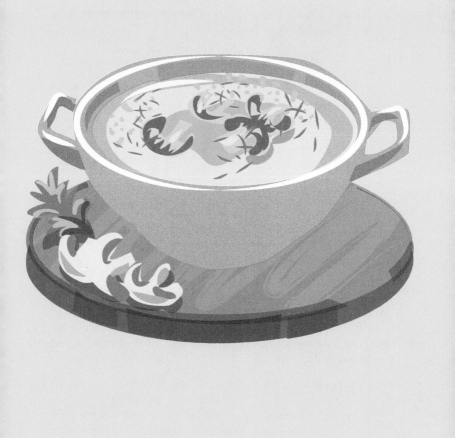

Diet //
The Macrobiotic Diet

Macrobiotic Diet

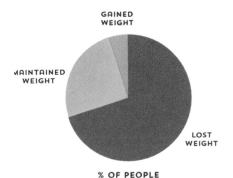

GAINED
WEIGHT

MAINTAINED
WEIGHT

LOST
WEIGHT

% OF PEOPLE

BY THE NUMBERS
**Fitness Statistics:
of the 100 peple we contacted**

 10% recommended
daily exercise in
order to see results

 48% saw weight loss
after 7 days w/o exercise

 5% would not
recommend it

DON'T EAT:
**Fast food and packaged high-sodium
foods, like chips, French fries, and cookies.**

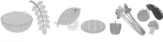

EAT:
**Focus on consuming whole grains, supplemented
by vegetables and other plant foods.**

The approach has been around for centuries, but the earliest mention of the term comes from Hippocrates, born in 460 BC in ancient Greece. He used the term to describe people who had great health, longevity, and practiced a simple, mostly vegetarian diet.

What's it for?

 Proponents say it will help you lose weight and be healthier. The diet, however, lacks good clinical studies to back the claim.

It might have cardiovascular benefits, since its focus is on whole grains, veggies and non-processed foods.

The macrobiotic diet is frequently suggested for people with cancer, but the American Cancer Society does not recommend it and believes it could do more harm than good.

 People who are sick, children, and pregnant women could possibly not get enough required nutrients on the macrobiotic diet.

How it Works:

1. You should only be eating "real" food that is organic, and preferably grown locally.

2. Whole grains should make up the bulk of your diet: brown rice, rye, buckwheat, barley and oats.

3. Vegetables and other plant products are also required, and shouldn't be frozen or processed.

4. Fruit, fish, seafood, and nuts can be eaten once or twice a week. Red meat, poultry, eggs and dairy should be absent or only rarely eaten.

5. You'll have to make sure you're still getting key nutrients that come from animal products, like vitamin B-12. Earlier versions of the diet recommended living on brown rice and water—a big no that could lead to nutritional deficiency.

Pros

👍 With more whole grains in your diet, you'll likely remain satisfied and full after meals.

👍 You'll be eating less processed food, which is always good for overall health.

👍 It should be fairly effective at keeping your bad cholesterol and triglycerides low.

Cons

👎 It's not recommended by major medical groups and experts, who say that it relies heavily on carbohydrates.

👎 The risk of malnutrition is possible, especially if foregoing all animal products.

👎 You will need to avoid cooking with microwaves and possibly even pots and pans to stick to an all-natural diet.

👎 You'll have to dig to find macrobiotic recipes or create your own.

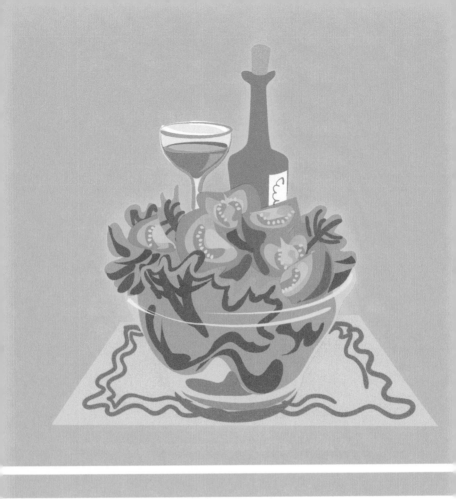

Diet //
The Mediterranean Diet

Mediterranean Diet

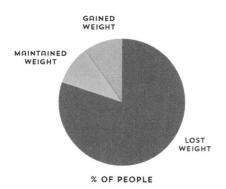

GAINED WEIGHT

MAINTAINED WEIGHT

LOST WEIGHT

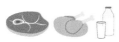

% OF PEOPLE

**Fitness Statistics:
of the 100 peple we contacted**

 85% recommended daily exercise in order to see results

 12% saw weight loss after 7 days w/o exercise

 10% would not recommend it

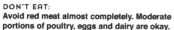

DON'T EAT:
Avoid red meat almost completely. Moderate portions of poultry, eggs and dairy are okay.

EAT:
Eat lots of fresh produce, whole grains and seafood. Flavor with olive oil, herbs and spices.

Who made it?

The diet consists of traditional cuisine from countries like Spain, Greece, Lebanon, and others bordering the Mediterranean Sea.

What's it for?

It's well-known that people bordering the Mediterranean have longer, healthier lives. They also suffer less from chronic and fatal diseases, like cancer and obesity.

How it Works:

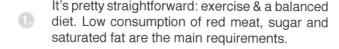

It's pretty straightforward: exercise & a balanced diet. Low consumption of red meat, sugar and saturated fat are the main requirements.

Other than that, just pick out some recipes you like. There isn't one "Mediterranean" diet, but both Greek and Spanish cuisines, for instance, share similar features—olive oil, fresh veggies, beans, flavorful herbs and seafood.

3. In general, you should be eating very little red meat and sweets. Wine can be consumed in moderation.

4. Fruits, veggies, grains, olive oil, and everything else fresh and plant related should be the main facet of your meals.

5. Fish and seafood should be your primary protein source and eaten at least twice a week.

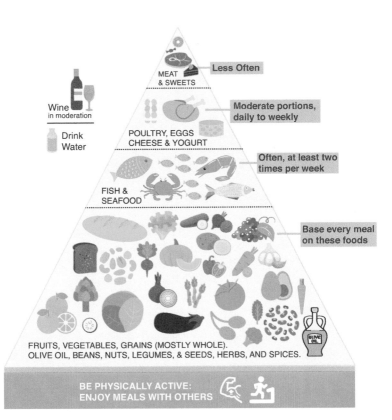

Pros

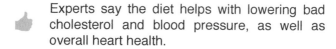 Experts say the diet helps with lowering bad cholesterol and blood pressure, as well as overall heart health.

It's less likely you'll have weight issues, especially if you're physically active.

The diet is safe for anyone and can be adjusted to dietary and religious restrictions.

You'll be meeting government health recommendations for fat, protein, carbohydrate and salt intake.

It offers a wide variety of meal choices, and recipes are easy to find online or in cookbooks.

Cons

While the foods you're eating will be good for you, they can still be calorie-rich. You'll have to count your calories if you're trying to lose weight. There are plenty of apps and online tools to help you keep track.

In the States, it's a moderately pricey diet. Olive oil, fresh fish, fresh produce and nuts can increase your grocery bill, but it's possible if you buy items on sale or grab some coupons.

Planning and cooking a good meal can be time consuming.

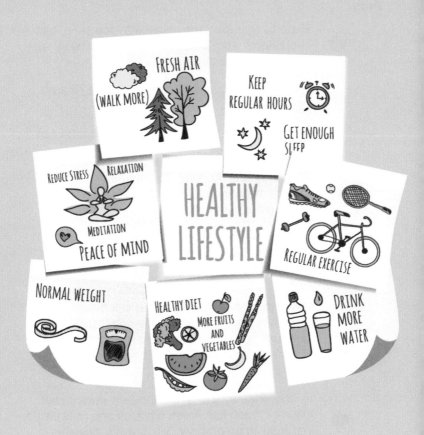

**CHAPTER 2 //
PROGRAMS**

How to Use This Section

Programs, unlike diets, are centered on pre-packaged meals that are complemented with activities, like weight-lifting, calisthenics, yoga and running. The pre-packaged meals can be supplemental shakes, mail-delivered foods and powders or a combination of both. They're advertised heavily and use celebrity endorsements.

Decide which program might be for you with these sections:

What Can I Eat?

Pretty straightforward. We tell you what the program requires you to eat.

Does It Work?

We tell you whether we think the program can give you results.

Break It Down!

You'll learn what each program is about & the reasoning behind it.

Weight
WATCHERS

What Can I Eat?

Just about anything. From pastas and steak to burgers and ice cream. There are no time blocks on when to eat or when not to eat, it's just about points. In its simplest form, each food is assigned a number of points based off how filling the food is.

Does It Work?

Yes. Their claim is 2 pounds a week, every week, and by that measure it might work better one week and not the next. But by implementing a point system that is methodical, there will be results.

Break It Down!

Essentially, it's a mathematical formula. The idea behind Weight Watchers is to aid members in losing weight by creating a positive environment. This environment is centered on meetings where smart eating habits, exercise routines and struggles are spoken about in an open forum.

The mathematical component of Weight Watchers comes into play in the menu. In the program no foods are off limit. You can eat anything you want so long as you stay within your calorie count. It's a point system that is compatible with other diet plans and as a result, can be very useful in losing weight.

When a member obtains their goal, the maintenance period begins. This is a six week time-frame where the member gradually adjusts their consumption and dietary habits to the point that a healthy weight is maintained for a prolonged period.

PLOT OUT YOUR GOALS -

 Make a blueprint for success by breaking your goal down into parts. Make a chart of the timeline and build it up, week by week, with details of shopping strategies, exercise tips and so forth.

ENVISION YOUR SUCCESS -

 Visualize yourself succeeding in particular scenarios, like making the right choices when dining out and think about how good you'll feel about achieving your goals.

DON'T SABOTAGE YOURSELF -

 Many of us unconsciously sabotage ourselves with self-destructive thoughts: "I'll never lose weight." Whenever you catch yourself thinking this way, try to substitute more constructive statements.

BE YOUR OWN CHEERLEADER -

 You wouldn't call a friend "fat" or "ugly," would you? You deserve the same respect, so try becoming your own best friend. Celebrate your progress.

AVOID BEING A PERFECTIONIST -

 Try not to think in all-or-nothing terms — that you've blown your diet, for example, simply because you've overdone it at one meal.

FOLLOW THROUGH WITH YOUR GOALS -

 You can't just think yourself slim, but you can think yourself into the right frame of mind to optimize your prospects.

AFFIRM YOUR SELF-BELIEF -

 Feel your confidence wavering? One way to reinforce your self-belief is with positive affirmations: simple, self-validating statements repeated as often as possible, preferably daily.

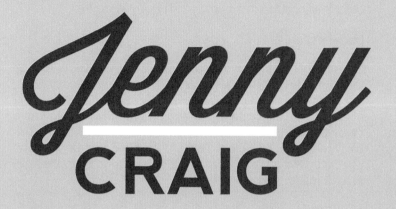

Programs //
Jenny Craig

What Can I Eat?

What they tell you. The program here is based around a pre-packaged plan and a consultant. The menu is designed based on your current health and your goals and your success really depends on how you handle structure.

Does It Work?

Yes and no. In the short term, yes. Even without attending the consultant meetings, just sticking to pre-packaged meals, the people we spoke to lost weight. However, the price tag makes it difficult to remain on the program. Ms. Craig has a study posted on the website from the Journal of the American Medical Association. This study states that on average people on the program lost about 10% of their overall weight in a 12 month period.

Break It Down!

There are a lot of packages that they offer, but the gist of them is pretty much the same.

The plans include their pre-packaged meals, which are very low in calories, the personal consultant that is there to guide you, answer any questions and keep you motivated and the online tools that is meant to simplify the entire process.

In theory, there are no "off-limits" foods on Jenny Craig. The way the plan is set up, you eat from the pre-packaged (usually 1200 calories a day) foods throughout the day and as the weight begins to fall off, the consultant allows you to begin to eat outside the pre-packaged food. It is here that the plan tries to educate the consumer on how to shop, cook and eat in a healthier manner.

Jenny Craig
CONSULTANT AND YOU DYNAMIC
1ST MEETING

---

1. **ASK YOUR CONSULTANT QUESTIONS**
ABOUT HOW BEST TO WORK TOGETHER

2. **REVIEW YOUR CURRENT WEIGHT AND**
SET REALISTIC GOALS YOU'LL ACHIEVE TOGETHER

3. **PLAN OUT YOUR STRATEGY**

4. **FEEL SUPPORT WHEN YOU REALIZE**
YOUR CONSULTANT IS THERE FOR YOU EVERY STEP OF THE WAY

5. **ENJOY A POSITIVE, CARING ENVIRONMENT**

6. RELAX AS YOUR CONSULTANT EXPLAINS THE PROCESS

7. INDULGE YOURSELF AS YOU AND YOUR CONSULTANT
CHOOSE YOUR JENNY CRAIG MEALS
FOR THE UPCOMING WEEK - THESE ARE DESIGNED
TO HELP YOU **LOSE AN AVERAGE OF 1-2 LBS/WEEK**

Nutrisystem

What Can I Eat?

What they tell you. Nutrisystem and their plethora of celebrity success stories all swear by the program of eating only what they ship to your door, as well as avoiding alcohol and dining out. The people we contacted all seemed to really, really support it.

Does It Work?

With all the Hollywood endorsements, you're probably expecting miracles, right? Wrong. Those same people who loved it for its simplicity also warned us that if you do not supplement the diet with lots of fruits, yogurts, nuts, salads and other healthy snacks, you end up plateauing.

Break it Down!

When it comes to Nutrisystem, you don't have to look past the meal plans. They include a collection of options that keep to a 50% carbs, 25% protein and 20% fats and 5% other. Their carbs, however, are good for you. They call them "smart carbs," which do not raise blood sugar to the levels that other carbs do. So certain fruits, bread and rice are off limits. If you stick to the calorie limit they suggest, you eat the plans they ship, and you supplement with their healthy suggestions, you will lose anywhere from 2-5 pounds a week.

Nutrisystem
THE AVERAGE

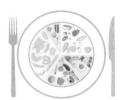

	BREAKFAST AVERAGE	LUNCH AVERAGE	DINNER AVERAGE	DESSERT/SNACK AVERAGE
CALORIES	160	200	240	145
FAT	4g	5g	7g	5g
CHOLESTEROL	11mg	11mg	30mg	7mg
SODIUM	220mg	440mg	520mg	150mg
CARBS	25g	30g	30g	20g
FIBER	4g	4g	3g	4g
TOTAL SUGAR	8g	5g	4g	8g
PROTEIN	7g	11g	16g	6g

Slim-Fast

What Can I Eat?

Whatever you are making for dinner, as long as it is sensible. Slim-Fast is mainly concerned with what you DON'T eat for breakfast and lunch. As for dinner, they let you go wild. Their "wild" is defined as 500 calories, but there is no hard limit.

Does It Work?

Better than most, according to the people we spoke to. Nearly everyone who followed Slim-Fast's 3-2-1 plan saw a significant (4-6 pounds a week) weight loss while only exercising a couple of times a week at most.

Break it Down!

Slim-Fast currently sells itself as a 3-2-1 dietary supplement. It's three 100 calorie Slim-Fast snacks enjoyed throughout the day, two meal-replacing Slim-Fast shakes and one free meal. It's very simplistic, straightforward and surprisingly successful.

SLIM-FAST

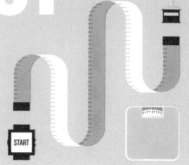

GETTING STARTED!
How do I know if I am ready to start losing weight?

Do you want to lose weight because YOU want to, and not because someone else thinks you should?

Do you feel enthusiastic about making a personal commitment to "why I can", rather than the "why I can't"

Are you willing to explore ways to incorporate regular physical activity into your daily life?

Do you think of losing weight and living a healthy lifestyle as an investment in your future as well as an investment in the "now"?

Answering "Yes" to these questions shows that you have a positive "can do" attitude that will go a long way in helping you get started on your weight loss journey.

Biggest
LOSER

What Can I Eat?

A bunch of small healthy meals throughout the day. Nearly 45% of the food you consume is lean protein, followed by a strong amount of low-fat dairy or soy, fruits and vegetables, whole grains, beans, and nuts.

Does It Work?

If you are willing to sweat it out and spend some time reading, you will see results. The idea is that you eat to rebuild and refuel. If you are not working out, the excess protein could become excess weight.

Break It Down!

The concept of these continuous small plates comes from the hit TV show's 4-3-2-1 Pyramid. Like Slim-Fast, the numbers here represent servings that you consume throughout the day. It's four servings of fruits and vegetables, three servings of lean protein, two servings of whole grains, and 200 calories of "extras."

THE BIGGEST LOSER

HOW THEY DID POST TV

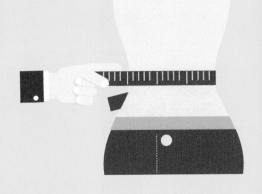

SEASON	CONTESTANT	WEIGHT LOSS ON THE TV SHOW	LAST REPORTED WEIGHT
1	Ryan Benson	**- 122** lbs	**+ 90** lbs
2	Kelly Miner	**- 79** lbs	**- 22** lbs
4	Bill Germanakos	**- 164** lbs	**+ 37** lbs
5	Ali Vincent	**- 112** lbs	**+ 20** lbs
7	Helen Phillips	**- 140** lbs	**+ 18** lbs
12	John Rhode	**- 220** lbs	**+ 5** lbs
15	Rachel Fredrickson	**- 155** lbs	**- 5** lbs

Herbalife

What Can I Eat?

Pretty much anything that tickles your fancy. Herbalife is a brand of shakes, teas and bars that are meant to replace meals while providing all the nutrients your body needs.

Does It Work?

Not really. There are hundreds of success stories scattered throughout the web, but they all read like marketing ads. So you have to take these stories with a grain of salt, as Herbalife has a pyramid scheme aura to it. For every success story online, there are four or five concern stories about investing a lot of money and not really seeing results.

Break It Down!

The sales pitch and promise is similar to other diet programs: replace two of your meals with the shake and have about 4 liters of water daily – usually, via their branded teas. The claim is that the protein, vitamins and minerals will keep you energized, full and active as you burn fat throughout the day.

HERBALIFE

The Basics for Maintaining Good Nutrition

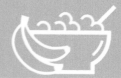

HEALTHY BREAKFAST

Start your day right! Breakfast is important because it kick-starts your metabolism and provides energy for you to use throughout your day.

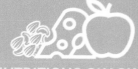

NUTRITIOUS SNACKS

Fruits, vegetables and small servings of protein – such as nuts, yogurt or low-fat cheese during mid-morning and mid-afternoon – help you avoid overeating at lunch or dinner time.

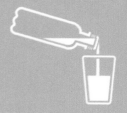

REGULAR HYDRATION

Ensure a regular intake of fluids to stay properly hydrated.

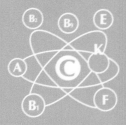

VITAMINS & MINERALS

These are an important part of a balanced diet needed to support your body's healthy functioning and metabolism

ESSENTIAL NUTRIENTS

Your body needs nutrients to function properly or your health will suffer. Getting the right amount of nutrients is called Balanced Nutrition. The nutrients known to be essential for human beings are proteins, carbohydrates, fats and oils, minerals, vitamins and water.

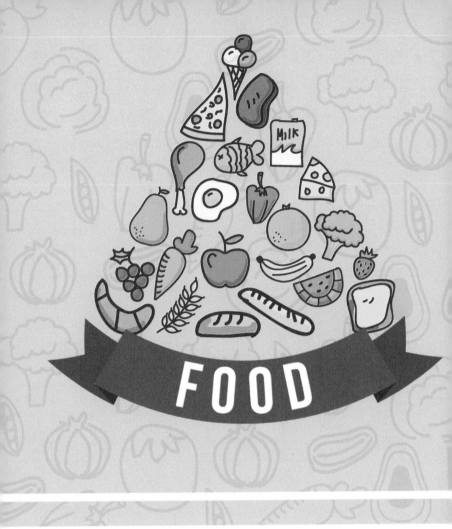

CHAPTER 3 //
Breaking Down the Food Pyramid

How to Use This Section

While the diets and programs earlier in the book all have different ideas about what makes up a "healthy" diet, here we turned to the science.

Nutrition Basics

This section is for giving you an idea of the basic components that your body needs to function. Whatever diet you choose, make sure it allows you to fulfill these essentials.

Top 10 Diet and Health Myths

Everyone thinks they know a few things about dieting, but what if they're actually wrong? A lot of conventional dieting wisdom misses the mark and acts against your goals.

Make Vegetables Work for You

It's almost a cheat to point this out, but pretty much every diet has the same premise: eat more vegetables. Since hardly anyone's favorite food is broccoli, we'll try to help you make it part of your routine.

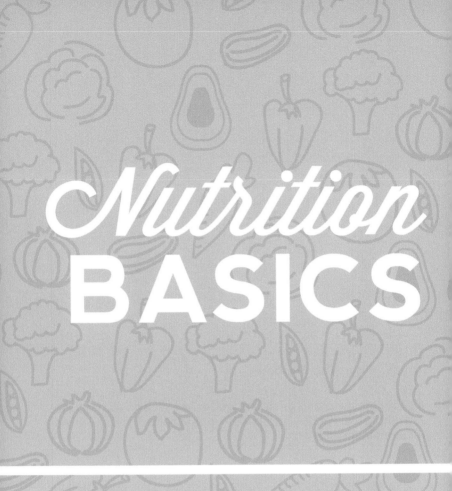

Nutrition
BASICS

**Breaking Down the Food Pyramid //
Nutrition Basics**

Whant do you need to eat to survive and thrive? What foods are going to kill us? Can you only eat salads to be healthy? Various medical professionals, health experts and diet gurus are still looking for answers to these questions, but for now, it's best to just stick to the basics. When picking a diet, try to make sure it will help you meet these dietary recommendations.

Water //

It's what your body's made of, so drink a lot of it—as in 2 liters of it. Ditch soda, juices and other sugary concoctions and consider them on the same level as dessert. If you're trying to lose weight, these calorie-rich drinks are only adding to your waistline.

Dietary Fat //

No, really, you need fat! The good kinds of fat contain essential nutrients, and your body uses fat to keep your body running. Still, your fat intake shouldn't exceed 30 percent of your daily calories.

There are the four different types of fat:

Saturated Fat:

You should only get 10% of your daily calories from this type of fat, so between 180-250 calories a day. It's found mostly in animal foods, e.g. milk, cheese and meat. Poultry and fish have less saturated fat than those foods. Also found in tropical oils like coconut oil and cocoa butter. Foods made with butter, e.g. cookies and cake, also have a lot of saturated fat.

Trans Fat:

Eat as little of this type of fat as possible. Trans fat has been changed by hydrogenation, which increases its shelf life and makes it harder. This hardness is good for crispiness in crackers and crusts. Processed foods, snack foods, cookies, some salad dressings, and food made with hydrogenated oils contain trans fats.

Unsaturated fat:

This is the main type of fat you should be eating. It comes in two forms—monounsaturated fat and polyunsaturated fat.

Monounsaturated fat:

Found in avocado, nuts, and vegetable oils (olive, canola and peanut). Eating these foods will help lower bad LDL cholesterol and keep your good HDL cholesterol high, but it's necessary to cut back on saturated fats.

Polyunsaturated fat:

Found in vegetable oils, such as corn, safflower, soybean, sunflower, and sesame oils. It is also the main fat in seafood.

There are two types of polyunsaturated fat:

Omega-3 fatty acids: Found in foods from plants like soybean oil, canola, walnuts, and flaxseed. Also found in fish and shellfish.

Note: A healthy diet should include 8 ounces or more of Omega-3 rich fish.

Omega-6 fatty acids: Found mostly in the liquid vegetable oils mentioned above.

Total fat:

This is how fat is labeled on food packaging. Food labels are not required to list the "good" fats, only saturated fat. Keep an eye out for high levels of saturated fat, and use this handy label guide:

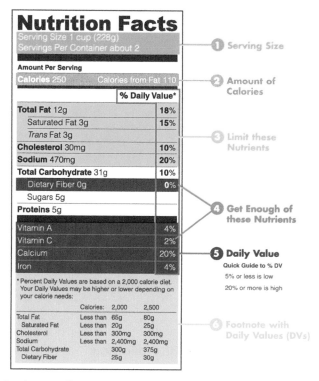

Carbohydrates //

Considered, as the "C" word in many diets, carbs get a bad rap. But you actually need some in a balanced diet. Your body uses carbs to make glucose, which give you fuel and keep everything in you running smoothly. It either uses the glucose or stores it for later use in your liver and muscles. Fruits, vegetables, bread, grains, and foods with added sugar all have carbs. The foods with added sugars (e.g.cakes, cookies and beverages) are the ones you want to avoid.

There are the two different types of carbs:

Complex carbohydrates //

Starch and dietary fiber are complex carbohydrates. Starch can be found in potatoes, dry beans, peas, and corn; while dietary fiber can be found in vegetables, fruits, and whole grain foods. You should get about 14 grams of fiber for every 1,000 calories you eat per day.

Dietary fiber is listed on food labels as either soluble fiber or insoluble fiber. You should be eating both, so eat a variety of foods.

Soluble fiber is found in the following:

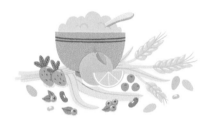

- Oatmeal
- Oat bran
- Nuts & seeds
- Most fruits
- Dry beans & peas

Insoluble fiber found in the following:

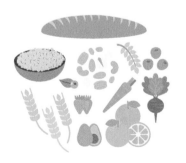

- Whole wheat bread
- Barley
- Brown rice
- Couscous
- Bulgur or whole grain cereals
- Wheat bran
- Seeds
- Most vegetables
- Fruits

Simple Carbohydrates //

This category includes sugars found naturally in foods like fruits and milk products. It also includes added sugars, the bad kind. They're added in food processing and don't have as many nutrients as foods with natural sugar.

Avoid added sugars listed in food labels by referring to the list below:

- Brown sugar
- Corn sweetener
- Corn syrup
- Dextrose
- Fructose
- Fruit juice concentrates
- Glucose
- High-fructose corn syrup
- Honey
- Invert sugar
- Lactose
- Maltose
- Malt syrup
- Molasses
- Raw sugar
- Sucrose
- Sugar
- Syrup

Protein //

The favorite category of many fad diets and diet products, protein is vital for a healthy body. You're made of proteins that are constantly being broken down to help you move about your day. They also need to be replaced. A sedentary adult man should eat about 2 ounces of protein a day, while a woman should eat 1.6 ounces. Overall, it should make up at least 10% of your daily calories, but not more than 35%. The numbers may vary slightly depending on your weight and fitness goals, so find out what's good for you.

Here are some examples that contain a good amount of protein

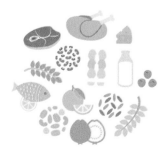

- Meats, poultry, & fish
- Legumes
- Tofu
- Eggs
- Nuts & seeds
- Milk & dairy products
- Grains, vegetables, & some fruits*

*(provide only small amounts of protein relative to other sources)

Types of Protein //

Complete protein:

 Foods that are complete proteins provide all the essential amino acids. Animal based foods are the best source—meat, poultry, fish, milk, eggs and cheese are high quality proteins.

Incomplete protein:

 Foods that are incomplete proteins are still okay to eat, but they don't contain all the essential amino acids. Eaten together, however, some of these can provide all the protein you need. For instance, rice by itself is missing some amino acids, but when paired with dry beans, you get a complete protein source.

Vitamins and Minerals //

A,B,C,D . . . K? Remembering which vitamins and minerals to consume can be daunting. The truth is, they can all easily come from a healthy diet and a multivitamin, if you want to be safe. Let's break it down for you.

VITAMINS & MINERALS

Both are essential for a healthy body and to prevent certain diseases.

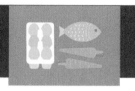

VITAMIN A

- Found in beta-carotene
- Promotes good eyesight
- Helps growth
- Healthy skin & tissue

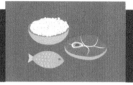

B VITAMINS

- B1- Thiamin
- B2-Riboflavin
- B3- Niacin- Helps release energy
- B9- Folic Acid-Important for pregnant women

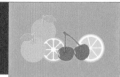

VITAMIN C

- Protects body from infections.
- Helps in absorption of calcium and iron
- Helps heal wounds

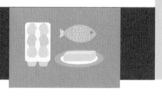

VITAMIN D

- Helps absorption of calcium for healthy teeth and bones

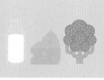

CALCIUM

- Strong teeth & bones
- Lack of calcium can lead to brittle bones (Osteoporosis / Rickets)

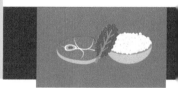

IRON

- Forms part of Hemoglobin
- Gives blood cells red color
- Lack of iron leads to anemia

And make sure to remember the more obscure minerals and vitamins:

Magnesium:

 Found in green veggies like broccoli and spinach, sunflower seeds, halibut, & whole-wheat bread.

Folic Acid:

 Found in grains, cereals, spinach, broccoli, legumes, orange juice and tomato juice.

Vitamin K:

 Found in cabbage, liver, eggs, milk, spinach, broccoli, kale and other green veggies.

Selenium:

 Found in meat organs, seafood, walnuts, and grain products.

Chromium:

 Found in meat, poultry, fish, cereals, nuts and cheese.

TLDR version—Eat your damn broccoli, kids.

TOP 10
Diet & Health
MYTHS

The Myth //

Don't eat after 6 p.m., 8 p.m. or whatever p.m.
Your mom or some other perpetually fit person may have told you this, but it's not true. You don't burn up food during the day and suddenly stop at night.

The Real Problem:

You're probably snacking at night and going way past your daily calorie limit with that tub of ice cream. If you can't ignore the craving, try going for a healthy option, like fruit. And don't starve yourself for hours at a time, it will only increase your chance of overeating.

The Myth //

It's okay to eat whatever, as long as you keep track of the calories.

It's really just the kind of food you're eating that's making you gain weight, not the amount. So, stick to eating healthy foods instead of trying to find loopholes to eating junk food again.

The Real Problem:

All food has calories, even the uber-organic locally-grown kind. Whole-wheat pasta and bread have just as many calories as their processed, unhealthy versions. Red wine and avocados are good for your heart, but they'll also add to your waistline. Keep track of your portion sizes to avoid the pounds piling up.

The Myth //

Eat many small meals throughout the day to boost metabolism.

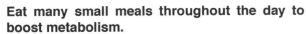

If you add fuel to your body's fire to keep it going, you won't slow down and let it gather up fat, right?

The Real Problem:

Food intake doesn't affect your metabolism much. If your metabolism is slow, part of the problem may be you're not fit enough. Build up some muscle or just exercise more to get your body to function better and burn more calories throughout the day.

The Myth //

Lose "X" number of pounds in "X" number of weeks or days.

This or that diet offers you a quick, unrealistic solution for your weight problem.

The Real Problem:

Unrealistic expectations are your enemy. The general rule is that one pound per week is the healthiest, most sustainable pace for losing weight. If you cut or burn 500 calories per day, it amounts to 3,500 calories per week, equivalent to one pound. It takes an hour every day of intense aerobic exercise to burn that amount.

The Myth //

Pasta makes you fat.

Pasta is a carb, and carbs make you fat.

The Real Problem:

You're not counting calories and probably eating half a box at dinnertime. Just a fist-sized portion of pasta is about 400 calories. If you want to get full without getting fat, you need to throw some lower calorie, stomach-filling foods on your plate, like veggies.

The Myth //

Always go for salad on a diet.

Salad will always be a lower-calorie option than any other meal, thanks to leafy green veggies.

The Real Problem:

Your salad may have lots of greens in it, but the toppings will get you. Shredded cheese, nuts, and dressings can send a salad's calorie count past double cheeseburger levels. Pay attention to the calories.

The Myth //

Milk is always good for you.

Milk has calcium. You need calcium. Milk moustaches are awesome. What's not to love?

The Real Problem:

All dairy, milk included, doesn't really have anything special to it. A few studies have found that people who ditched milk in their diet actually lost more weight. Others have shown it has no effect. If you really want milk and dairy, go low-fat, but there are other options for getting calcium.

The Myth //

You'll only lose weight on a diet.

You need some kind of structured plan to get you into the weight-loss groove.

The Real Problem:

Real weight loss requires long-term changes, not a short-term commitment. Whenever you stop the diet, the weight loss stops. Make changes you can actually live with and keep track of calories on a daily basis.

The Myth //

Cut back on calories—a lot—to really lose weight.

Eat less, weigh less.

The Real Problem:

This goes hand-in-hand with the previous myth. Unless you have a red-flag health issue, drastic changes are not your friend. Starving yourself will only make you miserable and more likely to end your dieting goals sooner. Go for an easy goal— cutting 250 calories a day—and you could possibly lose half a pound a week, or 26 pounds in a year.

The Myth //

"Light," "Diet," and "Fat-Free" foods are better for you.

It says "diet," right? Problem solved!

The Real Problem:

That fat-free cream cheese may be saving you a handful of calories per serving, but take a look at the nutrition label. Does it have more sodium? In order to get that diet junk to be edible, companies add a bunch of artificial sweeteners, sodium, and chemical additives that aren't good for you. Go for the real version, just eat it in smaller amounts.

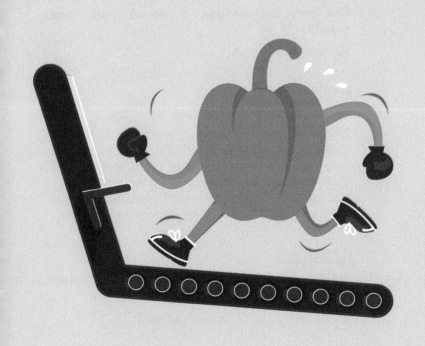

Breaking Down the Food Pyramid //
Make Vegetables Work for You

If the various diet plans, weight loss programs, and the nutritional section above haven't given you a clue: you need vegetables. The average American's plate today is a delicious mess of possibly organic cheese, grease and sugar with not a single green leaf in sight.

Let's do a little number comparison:

Food Consumption Per Capita
In 2004, the average American consumed

46
SLICES OF PIZZA

66.6
POUNDS OF BEEF

87.7
POUNDS OF CHICKEN

21.4
GALLONS OF MILK

31.2
POUNDS OF CHEESE

23.2
POUNDS OF ICE CREAM

31.2
POUNDS OF YOGURT

11.7
POUNDS OF CHOCOLATE

24.7
POUNDS OF TOTAL
CONFECTIONERIES

134
POUNDS OF FLOUR

These numbers have improved slightly in the past decade, but obesity is still at a level unheard of by even our grandparents. We're making slightly better choices, but soda is right on the heels of fruits and veggies as our fourth favorite food.

EATING MORE FRUIT AND SNACKS, LESS SALAD

Top 10 foods and beverages consumed **in-home** and **away-from-home**

2003 | 2013

#	2003		2013	
1	Sandwich	6.6%	Sandwich	6.8%
2	Soft drinks*	6.2%	Fruit	6.0%
3	Vegetables	5.8%	Vegetables	5.6%
4	Milk	5.8%	Soft drinks*	5.2%
5	Fruit	5.3%	Milk	5.1%
6	Coffee	4.6%	Coffee	4.6%
7	Fruit Juice	4.6%	Potatoes	4.0%
8	Potatoes	4.4%	Salty snacks	3.9%
9	Cold cereal	3.7%	Fruit juice	3.6%
10	Salads	3.4%	Cold cereal	3.5%

AGE-ADJUSTED PREVALENCE OF OBESITY AMONG U.S. ADULTS AGED 20-74

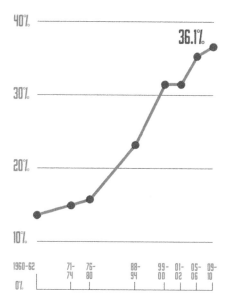

So how do you get yourself to like vegetables when they don't have the same flair as a burger with some fries?

Well, here are some tips to get those greens back in your diet:

1. You love bacon, but you really should be eating kale. Mix them together! A little cheese won't hurt either, but make sure your kale to cheese ratio is reasonable.

2. Avocado on a burger has the potential to decrease some bad effects of red meat.

3. Broccoli with mustard has the potential to improve its nutritional value. Cheese won't, but it's also a tasty option.

4. Mixing veggies with pasta or rice can make everything taste better.

5. Try a sauce, but make sure to find a healthy option, like pesto.

6. Smoothies are another way to get your veggie intake, and there are plenty of good recipes for throwing fruits in there, too.

7. Buy fresh veggies, not frozen ones, and add spices and herbs to bring out their flavor.

8. Look up recipes. Chances are you weren't born knowing what goes well with spinach, so use recipes to help you get more creative.

9. Once you figure out healthy meals you like, keep eating them. Don't make it a one- time thing.

DIET HACKS

SIMPLE, YET *creative*, THESE HACKS CAN HELP YOU START, ENJOY & STICK WITH YOUR DIETING JOURNEY. WHETHER YOUR *goal* IS MAJOR WEIGHT LOSS OR A HEALTHY HEART, HERE ARE *the best ways* TO ENJOY YOUR FOOD. WE OFFER SOLUTIONS FOR EACH OF THE SCENARIOS, FROM REPLACING FATTY FOODS *to keeping your diet on vacation.*

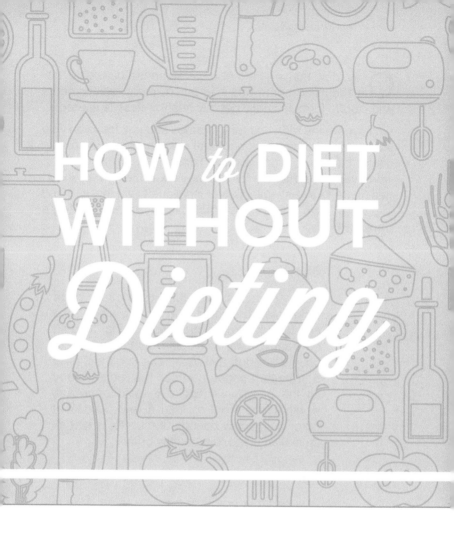

HOW to DIET WITHOUT Dieting

Diet Hacks //
How to Diet Without Dieting

Okay, now that we kind of understand the difference between good carbs and bad carbs, meal replacements and calorie formulas, let's get this healthy lifestyle started.

Let's ignore the fads and funky names and just focus on why you're even reading this book. All we want to do is provide useful information and simple tidbits to a healthier life... whatever a healthier life for you may be. Based on our inquiries made to a vast collection of individuals, via the web and in person, **here are the best Diet Hacks for maintaining a happier body.**

Start Early:

Eat breakfast. Maybe it's not a huge Colombian breakfast with beans, steak, rice and bread cakes, but eat something. It could be oatmeal with an apple on the side or a couple of eggs and toast. But don't just grab a drive-thru coffee and call it a meal. Nearly all the people we spoke to said breakfast, whether you want to lose a few pounds of fat or gain a few pounds of muscle, is just as crucial as sleep to a healthy body.

Against the Grain:

Low carbs is probably the way to go. Maybe you don't need to completely give up bread for all eternity, but cutting back on carbs seems to be a nice way to kick start a diet.

Muscle Building:

Don't ignore the protein. Whether it comes from a chicken breast or shiitake mushrooms (by the way, the greatest nickname you can give your vegetarian friends), protein is always tasty and, even better, always filling.

The Dark Knight:

Fiber. Although we are not always certain what it is, we do know we need more of it. The Common Denominator: Water and tea. These fluids, which in general are anti-sugar, anti-processed and most importantly anti-budget are a great way to shed a few pounds.

Snack Intelligently:

We all get cravings--some for ice cream, others for chips. The hack here is to make these snacks difficult to obtain. When you do eat ice cream or some chips, accompany it with a healthy snack, like a granola bar or fruit. Eat this healthy item first and that way you'll end up eating a smaller portion of the unhealthy craving.

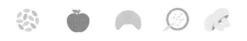

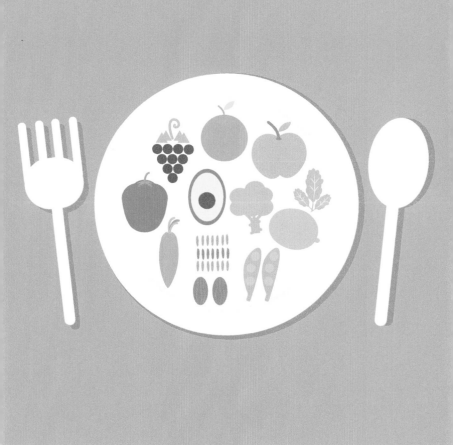

Diet Hacks //
How to Eat Your Veggies

For starters, regardless of our fitness goals, dream body or blood pressure, more veggies are always a good thing. So how can we go about simply eating a little healthier without our taste buds finding out? One of the simplest ways to accomplish this is by implementing what the internet calls: **This for That**. Pretty self-explanatory, just replace **This** not so great food with **That** healthier option that doesn't taste half bad.

Quinoa is the New Rice

 It doubles the protein of rice and has more than 150% of the fiber. Calories are a tad bit higher, but all in all it is a fair trade off.

Hold the Mayo

 If you want to eliminate hidden sugar & saturated fats from your diet, you can swap the creamy mayo for some silky mustard, which has neither.

From Coke to Tea to Water

 Another way to eliminate all that sugar is to switch all your soda intake to teas. Natural teas are not only sugarless, but they are packed with antioxidants. For those with massive coke cravings, try watering down the soda with ¼ water and gradually building up until the carbonation is a thing of the past.

Go Greek over Sour

 Sour cream is the bomb. Let's not kid ourselves. That stuff on top of a baked potato is amazing. But like all great joys in life, it isn't very good for us. Lately, we have been replacing our dollop of sour cream with a light Greek yogurt dollop. The taste is really good, a refreshing sour that comes with minimal calories and a hefty load of protein.

Bread Crumbs No More

 Chia seeds are like bread crumbs with protein, fiber and about half the sodium. Why we even use breadcrumbs is beyond our understanding.

Rehydrating the Hipster Way

 Sports drinks had their time, but in today's society they are a senseless collection of sodium and sugar. Coconut water is just as revitalizing and contains even more potassium than the top brands.

Got Almond?

 Almond milk is milk that tastes better than the regular stuff and has 6 times less sugar.

There are more foods that can be replaced with other foods. If you really want to go health-nut crazy, you might find yourself switching lettuce for kale, but the point is to just make small changes that have big results. Maybe almond milk isn't for you, but you end up loving quinoa. The only way to know is to try.

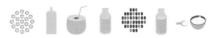

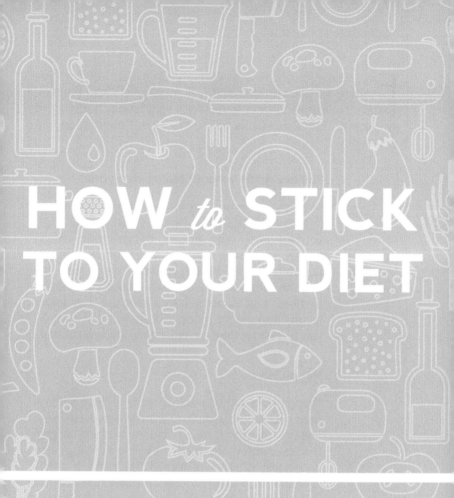

HOW *to* STICK TO YOUR DIET

Diet Hacks //
How to Stick to Your Diet

Fine, whatever, you're actually going on a diet. Let's get this started so you can quit and feel miserable about yourself before the weekend gets here. Well, maybe not. Let's try to avoid that. The Diet Hacks below are all set up to keep you on track.

Tell everyone without telling everyone.

Modesty goes a long way in anything you do in life. From dating to job hunting to dieting, if you're humble and modest, things might just go better. This isn't scientific or religious, it's just an observation. When you start your diet, tell your close friends and family about your hopes and fear that come with this journey. They might laugh, they might mock, but they might support you given that they do, you know, love you and all.

Happy Hour:

Going out to dinner, happy hour or a party is damn near impossible when you want to stay away from sodium, empty calories and tasty, tasty sugar. However, the West Coast movement of Veganism and going green has forced the hand of many restaurants to offer excellent healthy options. You can avoid the morning hangover and the empty calories of a night of drinking by volunteering to be the designated driver…and you might save a few lives – so good for you.

Trash the Scale:

The only thing worse than stepping on a scale while dieting is watching *Star Wars* Episode I, the Phantom Menace. Like the throwaway prequel, getting on the scale is not necessary, a little bit awkward and always humiliating. If you lost a few pounds you'll be happy only until the next time you weigh in and you only lost one pound. And if you gained weight, you might just quit...so don't bother with the scale. Instead, track inches on your body. Maybe you went down a pant size. The truth is, muscle and water weight affect the scale as much as fat, so only weigh in sporadically.

Fall in Love:

There are numerous studies online about dieting together. Type in #fitcouple into Instagram search and you'll find over 600,000 pictures assigned to it – so there has to be something to it. Prior to writing this book, we spoke to quite a few people (26 different guys and gals), who said they work out just a little bit harder when they go with a person they're attracted to. These same 26 also noted how when dining with people they are trying to impress (e.g. the cute girl from the subway, the scruffy barista from coffee breaks or the boss on a Tuesday lunch meeting), they limit the bad food and eat a lot of salad. And drink water. So if you're having a fat day, take your boss to lunch.

Take a Break:

If you've plateaued or you're just bored with your diet, try a little break. Take a couple of days off to eat what you love. Two things will happen after this 48 break.

1. You'll realize that these foods make you who you are, so you'll quit the diet on the spot, or

2. The more likely and beneficial option, you'll realize that eating healthy makes you feel so much better than salty chips and cheap soda. This moment of enlightenment will be just the little boost you needed to get back on your diet and continue towards a healthier life.

With all that considered, the greatest factor for sticking to a diet is simple: are you happy? Diets are hard, they're not fun and at times they can be hell. But with all that in mind, you should still be content. Maybe you're not seeing the results you pictured or maybe the lack of food is causing you to be irritable; but at the end of the day, if your diet is forcing you to go to bed frustrated, wake up annoyed, and spend the majority of the afternoon disgruntled, it might be time to change it.

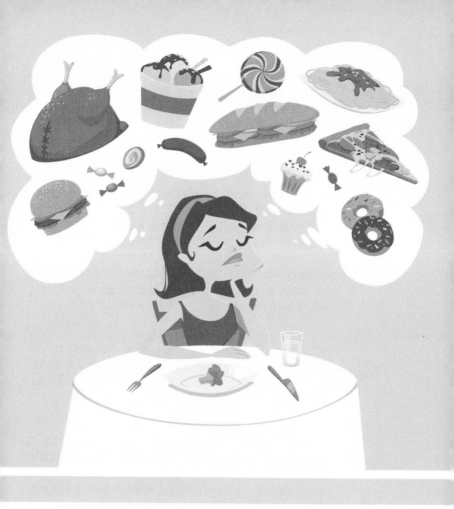

Diet Hacks //
How to Diet While Vacationing

Time away from the office, the emails, the rainy days…finally, a vacation. But with this adventure comes the burden of the diet. What do you do? You've been doing so well you've dropped a few sizes, you feel more energized and even your mother-in-law complimented you. But will this vacation ruin everything? Nope.

For starters, feel free to enjoy the comforts of vacationing to the fullest. If that means breakfast in bed, do it. But also consider that a vacation has a lot of time for unwinding and what better way to unwind than by doing some yoga on the beach, perhaps a light jog around the resort? Regardless of where you are staying, if you are active during your vacation, you are entitled to a few extra cocktails.

While we're staying active on our diet-cation, try using the stairs on your way back to the room. You'll burn a few extra calories in the chance that you poked around the dessert cart during dinner.

Whether vacationing with family or friends, see if you can get them to join in on the diet for the trip, it'll make the entire process a bit easier. Maybe you'll all agree to only having fruits while walking around Disney World, or while you're having dinner agree to go for a swim together upon returning to the hotel. These small, competitive activities make everyone participate and everyone support each other.

Always keep in mind that a vacation is the time to clear your body and mind. You're not spending hundreds, thousands even, to reinvent yourself. All you really want to do is relax for a few days. If you want to diet while traveling, more power to you, but if it is something that will make you miserable for the majority of the trip, well then maybe a dietcation isn't for you.

HOW *to* DIET
UNCONVENTIONALLY

Diet Hacks //
How to Diet Unconventionally

We'll we're at the end. If by now none of our hacks have hacked your waistline, sorry. But no worries, it isn't over. The internet is overflowing with the most obscure diets imaginable. There are more bizarre diets than there are characters in the Simpsons. **Here is our list for the top 5 obscure diets; hope one of them works!**

Sippin' on Gym and Juice:

Laid back, convenient and only moderately uncomfortable, the juicing diet is your typical fad. It spikes up anytime a celebrity posts a picture with a neon green smoothie or when FX marathons the Batman trilogy (go back and rematch the movies, Christian Bale drinks like seven of those throughout the three films). This fad diet basically requires two things: a blender and a gym membership. Simple enough, you liquefy your meals with the hope that you'll consume less of the beefier, pasty type foods and instead you'll reenergize your body with kale, leaks and other green things that puree easily. Some online say it should not be done for more than 48 hours, while others claim a few weeks. Our suggestion: give it a day, see how you feel.

The Cute Diet:

This diet feels more like a college party drinking game than a diet. There are a few online blogs that rave about it, while others see it as a joke. Either way, here it is. You only eat vegetables, but more specifically, vegetables with cute names. Cherry tomatoes, broccolini, baby carrots, chickpeas, etc. The logic behind it? Not much. It's just a fun, childish way to get children to eat more vegetables. Good luck with that.

"S" means NO!

There's some buzz going around that this might be the diet of the year, so prepare to be a cool kid by jumping on board first. The concept is don't consume salt, sugar, saturated fats, soda and snacks. Those promoting this diet claim that the removal of soda from your daily diet will result in more energy, controlling salt and sugar result in a healthier heart, and if you don't snack, you'll be more willing to eat your healthy vegetables and proteins during your meals.

Bi-Weekly:

Let's get funky. This is a trend that has been gaining some momentum across Europe, Australia and New Zealand. A bi-weekly diet consisted of an "on" week and an "off" week. During the "on" week you follow a strict diet of protein and fiber. There are no sugar, fats or carbs allowed. After the 7 day period you enter the "off" week. Here your diet returns to normal, you eat snacks, sweets and everything in between. However, you must exercise a minimum of 5 times within that week, for an hour each time. The idea is that gradually your body will begin to reject the negativity of sodas, fats and carbs while creating healthy habits of exercise and high quality meals. Additionally, the jumping back and forth allows you to stick with the diet given that there is a cheeseburger and pizza light at the end of the tunnel.

Gardening:

Simple and cute, the gardening diet asks that you grow your own vegetables. The hard work burns calories, the familiarity helps with nutrition control and because you raised them, you are more likely to consume them.

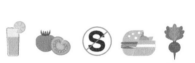

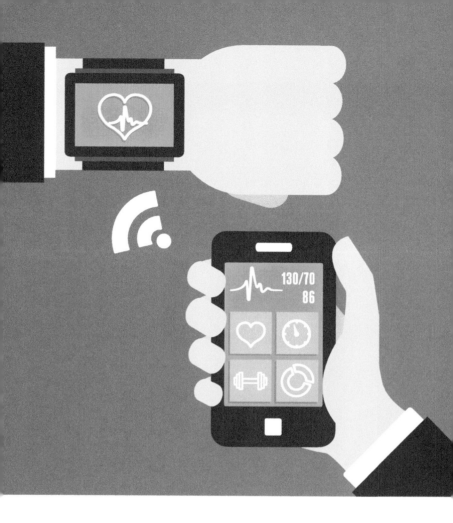

CHAPTER 5 //
Digitize Your Diet

Why work harder than you need to? We summarized four major tasks that are vital to keeping up with any of the diets and programs mentioned earlier. While somewhat daunting, they can be a breeze with a little help from your smartphone or computer. See which techie option is right for you.

There are several challenges to managing your diet and planning meals, and we've listed the biggest ones below—aided by technology. Let these intelligent machines do the hard work of losing weight for you. Well, just the parts with data. The rest is up to you.

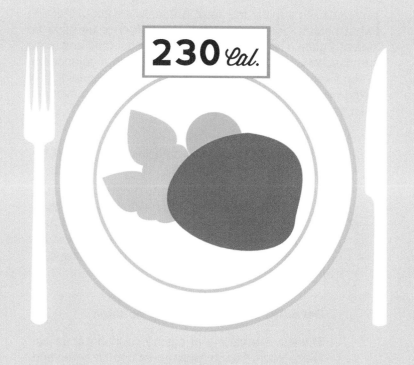

Food Tech //
Counting Calories

It sounds like a miserable task, but really it's about learning what healthy portion sizes look like. Most of us have no idea at a glance how many calories are in our food and we're surprised when we do find out. But achieving a balance between exercise and calorie intake is vital to maintaining or losing weight. It doesn't have to be a long-term commitment, but it's a good short-term learning tool.

Figure out how many calories you should be eating.

 The USDA's Choose My Plate program has a ton of resources on setting up a healthy diet. Use their Daily Food Plan calculator to get an idea of how many calories you need and how they should be distributed.(http://www.choosemyplate.gov/myplate/index.aspx)

Get a diet coach and calorie counter.

 There are a variety of calorie counting apps out there. Noom Coach (www.noom.com) is a free app that allows you to track the calories and foods you eat every day. It sets a calorie goal for you based on your weight goals and judges your foods as red (unhealthy), yellow (okay), and green (healthy). Noom Coach also includes a barcode scanner for easy input. MyFitnessPal and Lose it are two other good options.

Pay attention to nutritional info online.

 Many restaurants and chains make it difficult to find their calorie and nutritional info at their locations, but sometimes it's easily accessible online. While the apps mentioned earlier will usually have a match for your foods, sometimes it'll take some extra digging. CalorieKing (www.calorieking.com) offers extensive calorie information from nearly 300 restaurants and food chains.

HOW MANY CALORIES
DOES PHYSICAL ACTIVITY USE?

A 154-pound man (5' 10") will use up about the number of calories listed doing each activity below. Those who weigh more will use more calories, and those who weigh less will use fewer. The calorie values listed include both calories used by the activity and the calories used for normal body functioning.

MODERATE PHYSICAL ACTIVITIES:	IN 1 HOUR	IN 30 MINUTES
Hiking	370	185
Light gardening/yard work	330	165
Dancing	330	165
Golf (walking and carrying clubs)	330	165
Bicycling (less than 10 miles per hour)	290	145
Walking (3 ½ miles per hour)	280	140
Weight training (general light workout)	220	110
Stretching	180	90

VIGOROUS PHYSICAL ACTIVITIES:	IN 1 HOUR	IN 30 MINUTES
Running/jogging (5 miles per hour)	590	295
Bicycling (more than 10 miles per hour)	590	295
Swimming (slow freestyle laps)	510	255
Aerobics	480	240
Walking (4 ½ miles per hour)	460	230
Heavy yard work (chopping wood)	440	220
Weight lifting (vigorous effort)	440	220
Basketball (vigorous)	440	220

Food Tech //
Planning Meals

This is probably the hardest part of sticking to a diet. Why spend an hour cooking when you can simply sit in a drive-thru for five minutes? The truth is eating out makes it difficult to tell what you're eating, as many restaurants don't provide nutritional information. It's also more expensive than cooking for yourself.

Use a meal planner site.

Eat This Much (http://www.eatthismuch.com) will automatically plan all your meals for the day based on your daily calorie limit and other factors. The menu options include a few of the diets we mentioned, like Paleo, vegetarian and Mediterranean food. Recipes and nutritional content are included. The service is free, but has some paid features.

Get a planning service.

Cook Smarts (www.cooksmarts.com) is a paid monthly service, a bit like Netflix for your food. The service helps you plan out weekly meals based on your calorie and diet restrictions, provides cooking videos, new recipes every week, downloadable grocery lists and other food tutorials.

Get an app.

For organizing recipes you find online, the app Pepperplate is one good option for taking that mess of recipe links and putting them in an easy-to-access collection. ZipList is another good option that prepares grocery lists for you as well.

Find recipes.

There are dozens of recipe websites to choose from and you can organize them with the apps we mentioned above. But what if you're in a hurry and only have an egg, some ketchup and tuna in the fridge? Supercook (www.supercook.com) will give you recipes based on those ingredients, and will tell you what you're missing. The site Epicurious (www.epicurious.com) is one of the better recipe sites as it offers quick links to easy, low-calorie, low-fat, vegetarian and Mediterranean recipes. Their cooking blog offers a variety of information, including a weekly meal planner.

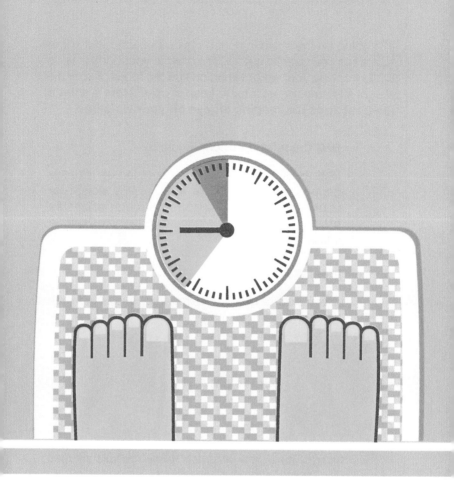

Food Tech //
Track Your Weight

Getting on the scale is no fun task for anyone, but sometimes you need to get an idea of what your body is up to. While tracking your weight shouldn't be the focus of your diet plan, it's an important factor to keep in mind. **Here's a list of the best apps for keeping an eye on your waistline.**

BMI Calculator (iPhone/Android) –

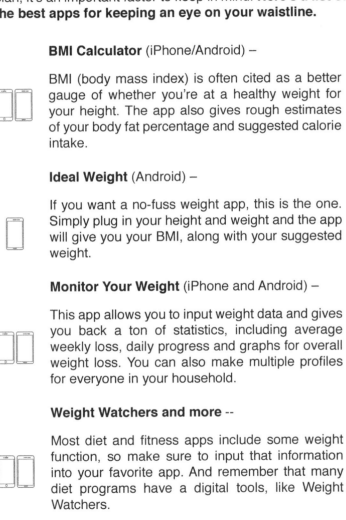

BMI (body mass index) is often cited as a better gauge of whether you're at a healthy weight for your height. The app also gives rough estimates of your body fat percentage and suggested calorie intake.

Ideal Weight (Android) –

If you want a no-fuss weight app, this is the one. Simply plug in your height and weight and the app will give you your BMI, along with your suggested weight.

Monitor Your Weight (iPhone and Android) –

This app allows you to input weight data and gives you back a ton of statistics, including average weekly loss, daily progress and graphs for overall weight loss. You can also make multiple profiles for everyone in your household.

Weight Watchers and more --

Most diet and fitness apps include some weight function, so make sure to input that information into your favorite app. And remember that many diet programs have a digital tools, like Weight Watchers.

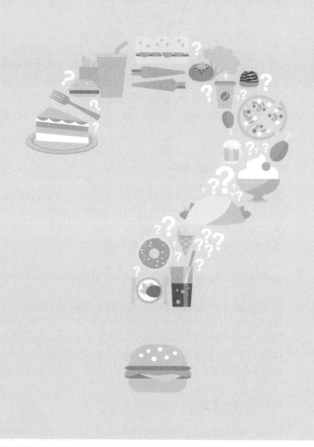

Food Tech //
Know What's in Your Food

It's pretty boring to read food labels all the time, but they're vital to getting the full scope of your food intake and needs. While a small cheeseburger and a salad may have the same amount of calories, it's likely that the latter is a better choice. Here are several good options for pulling up nutritional information on your daily meals.

Fooducate (iPhone/Android) –

This app focuses on pulling up nutritional information based on barcodes. The app displays a letter grade from A to D for each food, and presents the nutritional info in a more accessible way.

Calorie Counter PRO (iPhone/Android) –

Don't let its name fool you, this app is much more than a simple calorie counter. It's a comprehensive food scanner, allows you to log your nutritional intake, and it tracks your exercise. You can track up to 45 different nutrients.

MyFitnessPal (iPhone/Android) –

We mentioned this one earlier as a good calorie counting tool, but it also provides nutritional content for your foods and helps you keep track of what you're eating with a food diary.

HealthyOut (iPhone/Android) –

If you really don't have time to cook, HealthyOut can help you find a decent meal that won't hurt your diet plan. When available, you can view detailed nutritional information before you hit the restaurant or order delivery.

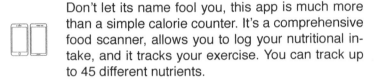

A NOTE FROM THE AUTHORS

The internet is overflowing with even more obscure and creative diets, like the all French fries diet or the video game diet. Whichever diet you pick, try to enjoy it and keep it simple. We'll all struggle with our image, our weight and our health. All we can do is educate ourselves, and try our best to have a good time living life. So all the best on your diet journey!

DATA SOURCES

http://www.weightwatchers.com/util/art/index_art.aspx?tabnum=4&art_id=48871&sc=3046

http://www.jennycraig.com/site/how-it-works-alt

http://content.nutrisystem.com/pdf/downloads/MealAverages.pdf

http://www.hsph.harvard.edu/nutritionsource/top-food-sources-of-saturated-fat-in-the-us/

http://www.clivir.com/pictures/vita/vitamin.jpg

http://oldwayspt.org/sites/default/files/images/Med_pyramid_flyer.jpg

http://oldwayspt.org/sites/default/files/images/Asian_pyramid_flyer.jpg

OTHER SOURCES

http://forum.lowcarber.org/forumdisplay.php?f=143

http://www.southbeachdiet.com/diet/

http://www.mayoclinic.org/healthy-living/weight-loss/in-depth/south-beach-diet/art-20048491?pg=2

http://www.diabetes.co.uk/forum/threads/vivs-modified-atkins-diet.18803/

http://www.atkins.com/Program/Phase-1.aspx

http://www.mayoclinic.org/healthy-living/weight-loss/in-depth/atkins-diet/art-20048485

http://forums.menshealth.com/topic/paleo-diet

http://thepaleodiet.com/the-paleo-diet-premise/

http://forum.bodybuilding.com/showthread.php?t=143796121

http://www.zonediet.com/why-zone/

http://www.livestrong.com/article/280370-the-pro-cons-of-the-zone-diet/

http://www.3fatchicks.com/forum/la-weight-loss/108369-volumetrics.html

http://www.livestrong.com/article/207333-volumetrics-diet-food-list/

http://www.veganforum.com/forums/showthread.php?28572 -raw-food-diet-Advice-Results

http://www.webmd.com/diet/raw-foods-diet

http://www.veganforum.com/forums/showthread.php?31471-Vegan-weight-loss

http://wellescent.com/health_forum/thread-1036-how_fast_does_the_dash_diet_work-diet_and_nutrition_with_high_blood_pressure.html

http://www.imamother.com/forum/viewtopic.php?t=117930

http://weight-loss.fitness.com/threads/34413-The-crude-Asian-diet-weightloss-journal

http://curezone.com/forums/am.asp?i=378594

http://www.3fatchicks.com/forum/sonoma-diet-mediterranean-diet/270404-sonoma-vs-mediteranean-diet.html

http://www.myfitnesspal.com/topics/show/1329718-does-weight-watchers-work

http://www.3fatchicks.com/forum/packaged-meals-clinics-nutrisystem-medifast-jenny-craig-etc/144765-jenny-craig-forum.html

http://www.webmd.com/diet/jenny-craig-diet

http://www.city-data.com/forum/diet-weight-loss/731054-anybody-nutrisystem.html

http://health.usnews.com/best-diet/slim-fast-diet

http://www.myfitnesspal.com/topics/show/465539-anyone-else-lose-weight-with-slim-fast

http://www.webmd.com/diet/biggest-loser-diet

http://www.nbcnews.com/business/business-news/many-herbalife-recruits-lost-money-dashed-dreams-f1B7899747

http://products.herbalife.com/

http://www.healthhabits.ca/2011/12/17/10-really-good-diet-hacks/

http://www.swansonvitamins.com/blog/natural-health-tips/food-replacement-hacks

http://www.veganforum.com/forums/showthread.php?31471-Vegan-weight-loss

http://wellescent.com/health_forum/thread-1036-how_fast_does_the_dash_diet_work-diet_and_nutrition_with_high_blood_pressure.html

http://www.imamother.com/forum/viewtopic.php?t=117930

http://www.hsph.harvard.edu/nutritionsource/top-food-sources-of-saturated-fat-in-the-us/

http://www.choosemyplate.gov/myplate/index.aspx

http://health.usnews.com/best-diet

http://www.webmd.com/diet/

http://www.mayoclinic.org/healthy-living/weight-loss/basics/diet-plans/hlv-20049483

http://weight-loss.fitness.com/threads/34413-The-crude-Asian-diet-weightloss-journal-)

http://curezone.com/forums/am.asp?i=378594

http://oldwayspt.org/

http://www.3fatchicks.com/forum/sonoma-diet-mediterranean-diet/270404-sonoma-vs-mediteranean-diet.html

http://www.clivir.com

http://www.eatthismuch.com

www.cooksmarts.com

www.supercook.com

www.epicurious.com

CPSIA information can be obtained at www.ICGtesting.com
Printed in the USA
BVOW10s2357090315

390722BV00006BA/14/P